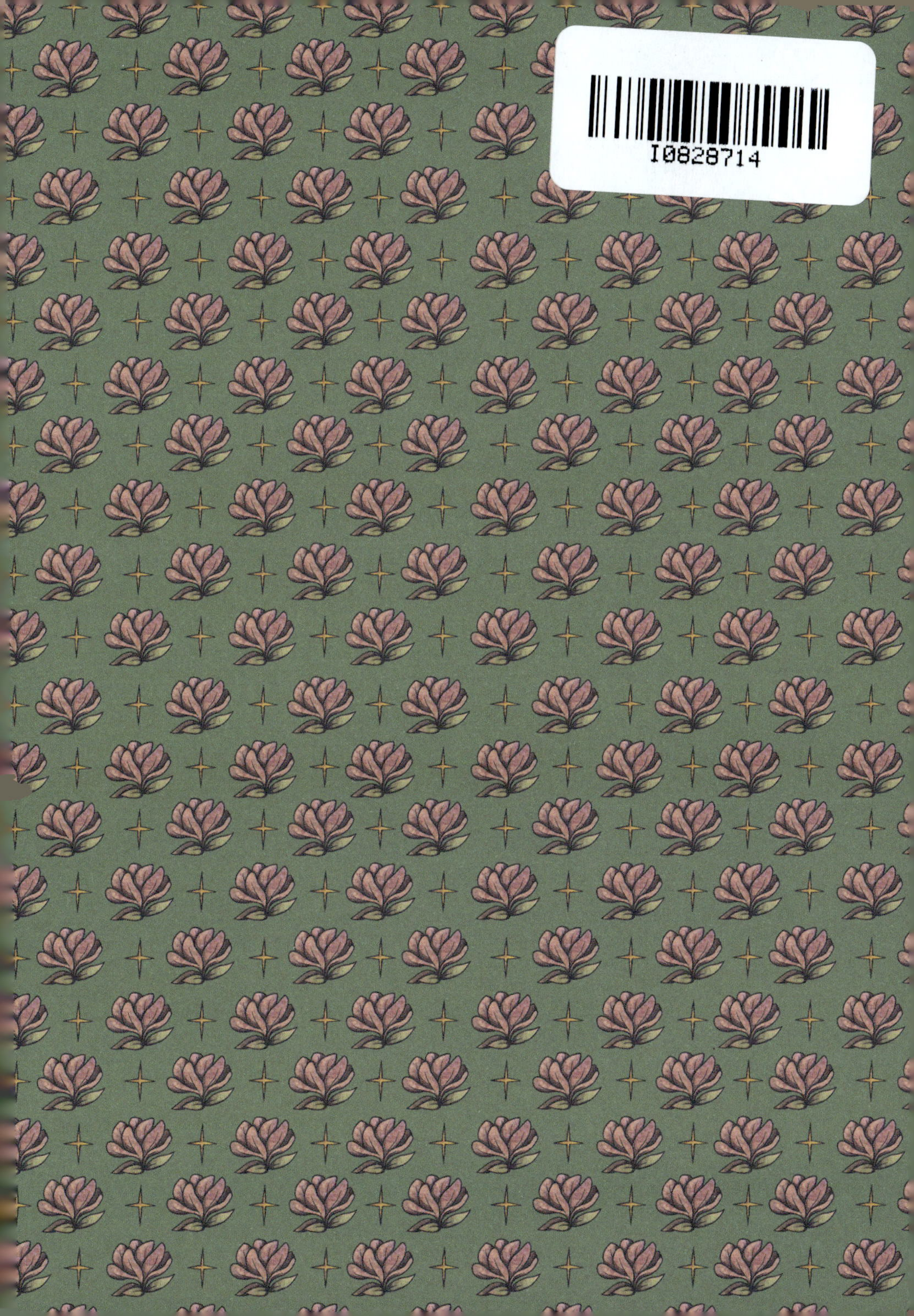
I0828714

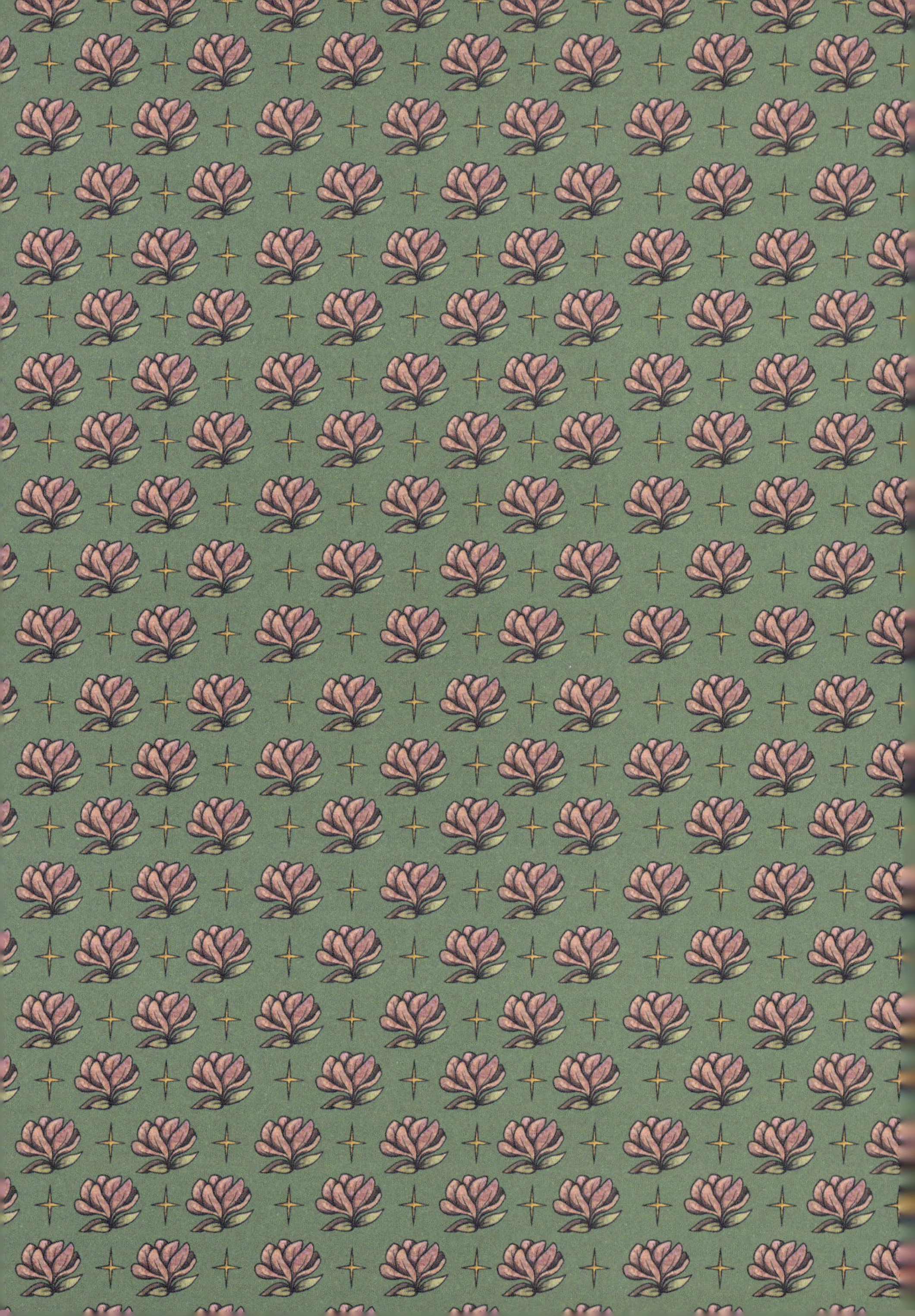

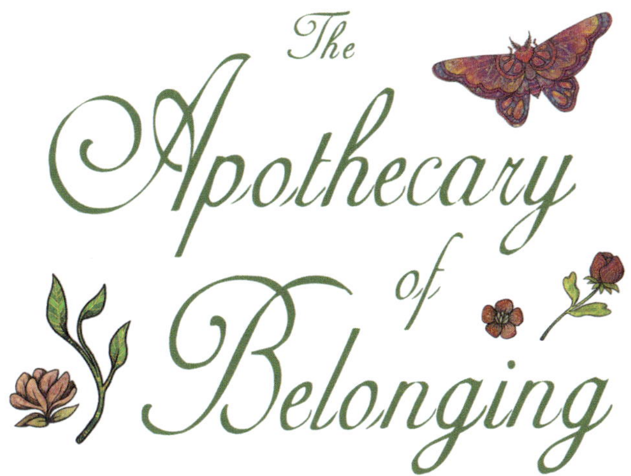
The
Apothecary
of
Belonging

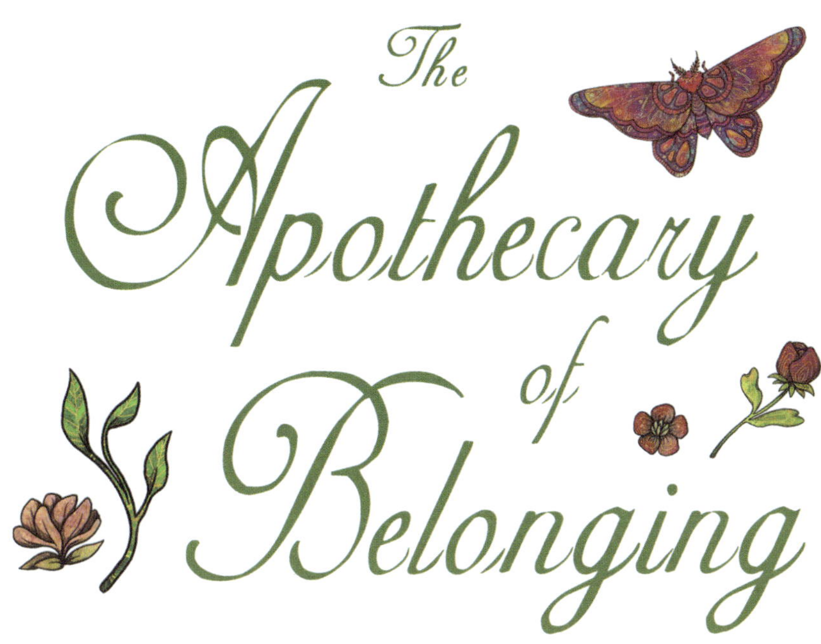


# The Apothecary of Belonging

## SEASONAL RITUALS & PRACTICAL HERBALISM

*reconnecting to the land, our bodies & our communities*

ALEXIS J. CUNNINGFOLK

foreword by
ARIN MURPHY-HISCOCK

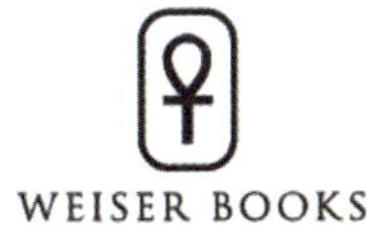

WEISER BOOKS

This edition first published in 2025 by Weiser Books, an imprint of
Red Wheel/Weiser, LLC
With offices at:
65 Parker Street, Suite 7
Newburyport, MA 01950
*www.redwheelweiser.com*



ISBN: 978-1-57863-882-6
Library of Congress Cataloging-in-Publication Data available upon request.
Interior images by Maryna Serohina/Ink Stories via Creative Market

Printed in China
WM
10 9 8 7 6 5 4 3 2 1

This book contains advice and information relating to herbs and plants and is not meant to diagnose, treat, or prescribe. It should be used to supplement, not replace, the advice of your physician or other trained healthcare practitioner. If you know or suspect you have a medical condition, are experiencing physical symptoms, or if you feel unwell, seek your physician's advice before embarking on any medical program or treatment. Readers using the information in this book do so entirely at their own risk, and the author and publisher accept no liability if adverse effects are caused.

*with all my love to the littlest trees of the loveliest grove*

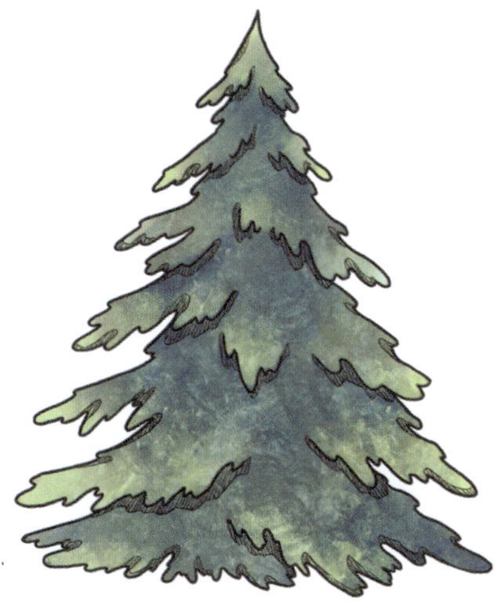

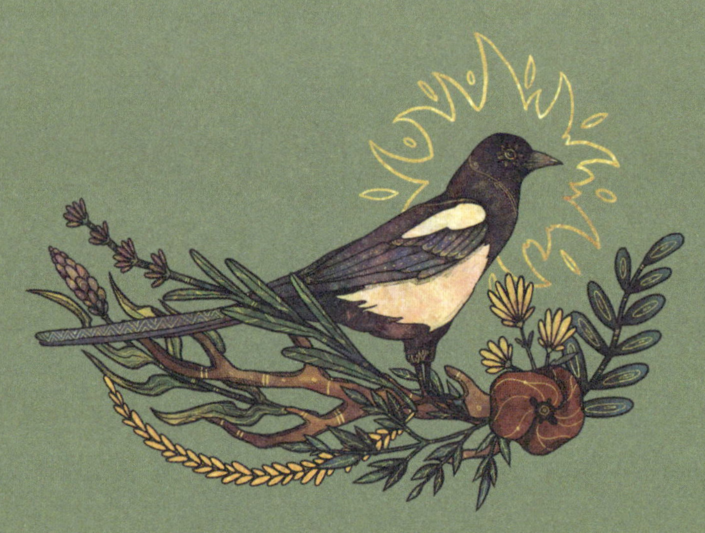

# Contents

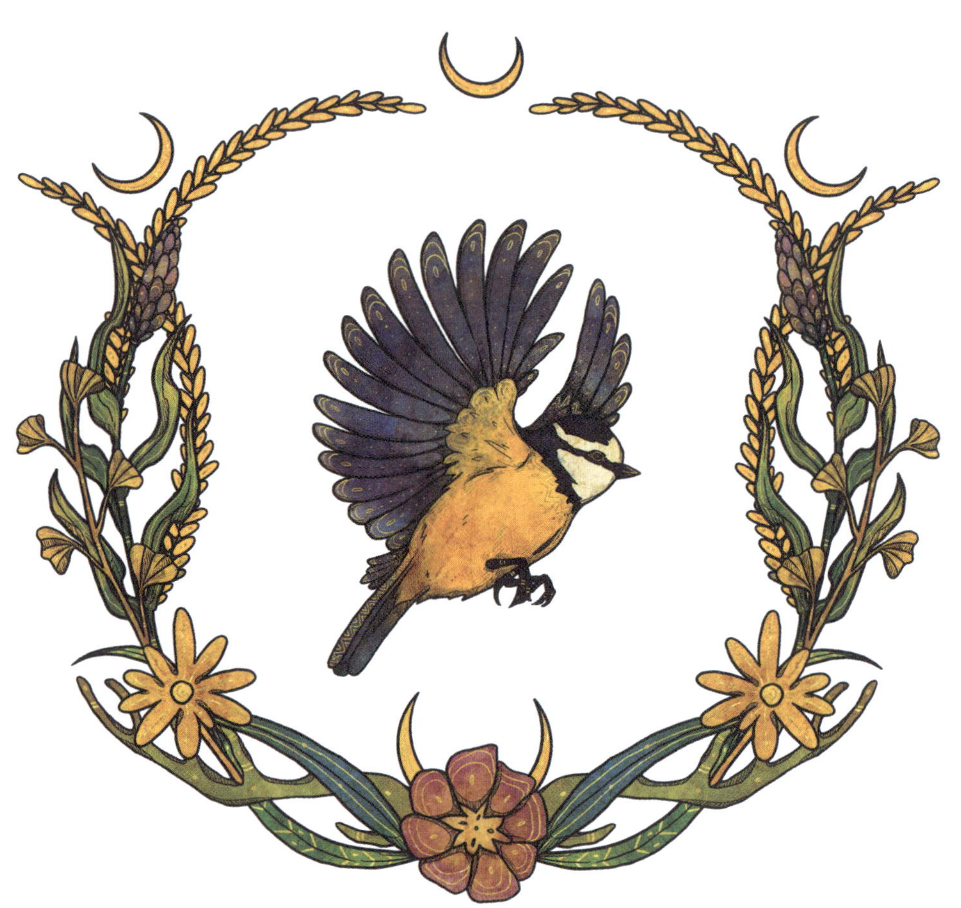

# Foreword

Walking a nature-based spiritual path means intentionally opening yourself to so many energies. It means reaching out to make connections with land, people, plants, trees. It means allowing yourself to be vulnerable to what they have to give, to share, and to communicate. It also means opening your eyes to the allies you interact with on a daily basis, learning how to acknowledge and reframe them in a way that becomes both respectful and mutually enriching.

In this book, Alexis explores the concept of interdependency. The energies and livelihoods of people, plants, and the earth are intertwined; they aid and support one another. Or, sadly, undermine or drain one another in times of imbalance . . . which seems to be all too often in these times of environmental and social crisis. Alexis teaches us that everything is woven together, from the herbs and plant allies to the psyches of those calling on them to the community at large moving around and through them to the land that nourishes and grows them. This also extends to time. The ancestors of the plants we know and use today, the many generations of people who lived and worked the land that we live on, the land that produces the plants we use medically and metaphysically . . . all these are entwined in the energies we encounter and interact with. This truth is both humbling and empowering.

It brings the concept of experience into a new light. Learning from experience—ours or that of others, ancestral or contemporary—is critical because it enables us to improve how we approach the next part of the ongoing cycle. Improving how we belong and how we facilitate others' belonging is crucial to our development as spiritually aware and literate people.

This book is a wonderful treatise on how we can call on the energies of herbs in a holistic fashion, drawing on them to supplement lack or deficiency in the context of wellness magically and physically. With her experience and training, Alexis has created an excellent intersection of medicine and magic, looking at how the physical intersects with the metaphysical. Everything is interdependent. Nothing exists in isolation. It is a truly holistic book that reminds us of how our work is always intersectional: When we work for ourselves, we also work for our plant allies, and for our community.

—Arin Murphy-Hiscock, author of *The Green Witch*

# Land Acknowledgment

I begin with honoring the lifeblood of the land—the two rivers cradling the valley I live in—and all the land that raised me, that I have lived with, and that I have traveled through.

I acknowledge and honor the Nisenan and Miwok as the traditional and living stewards of the land that I reside with and give respect to their Elders past, present, and becoming. I am grateful to be living with and learning from this land, and I acknowledge the resilience of Indigenous peoples, our complex history, and the deep need for repair, rematriation, and reconciliation.

This acknowledgment is a small part of my ongoing effort through word and deed to support the continuity of Nisenan, Miwok, and Indigenous ancestral traditions and future dreamings.

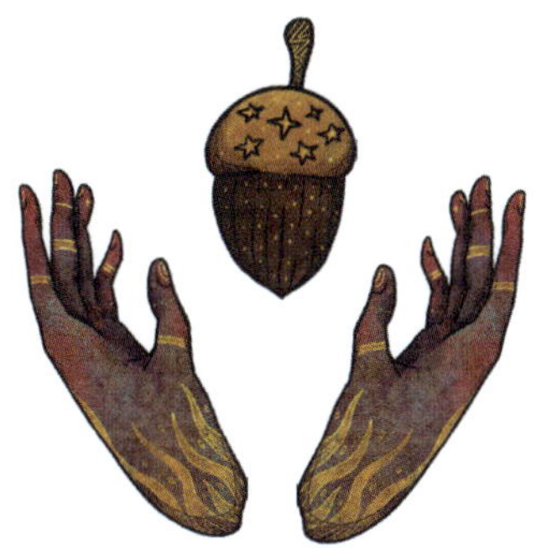

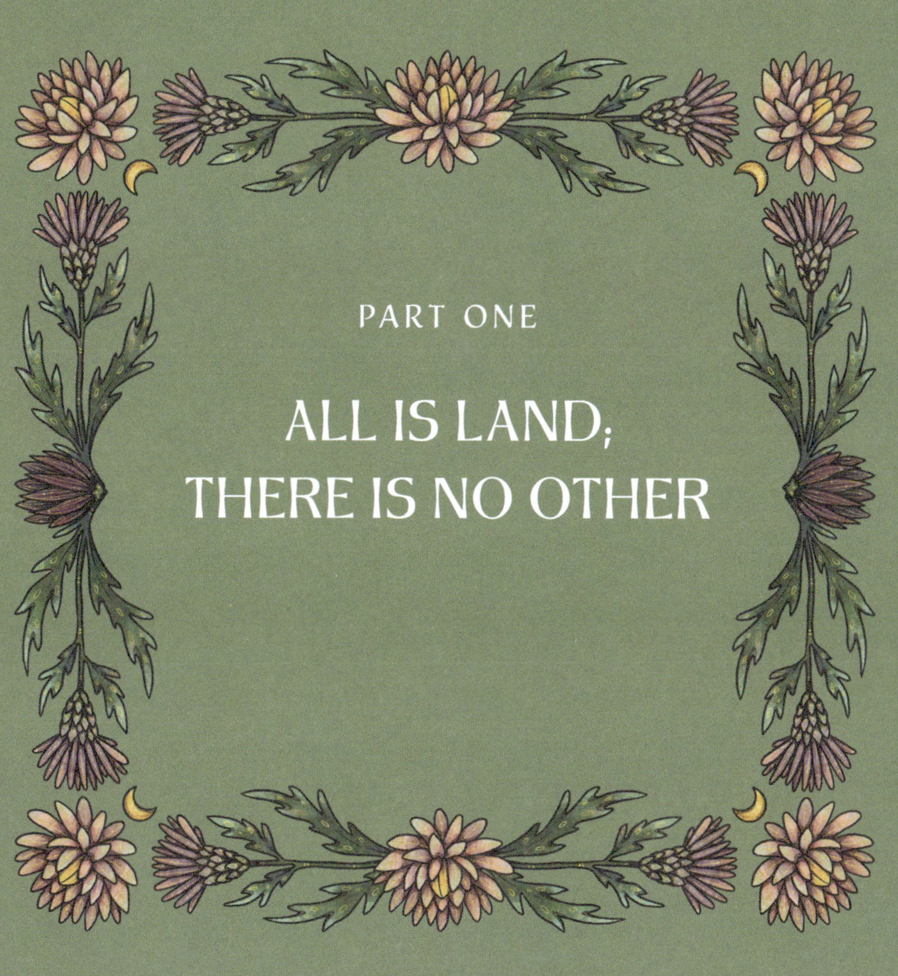

PART ONE

# ALL IS LAND; THERE IS NO OTHER

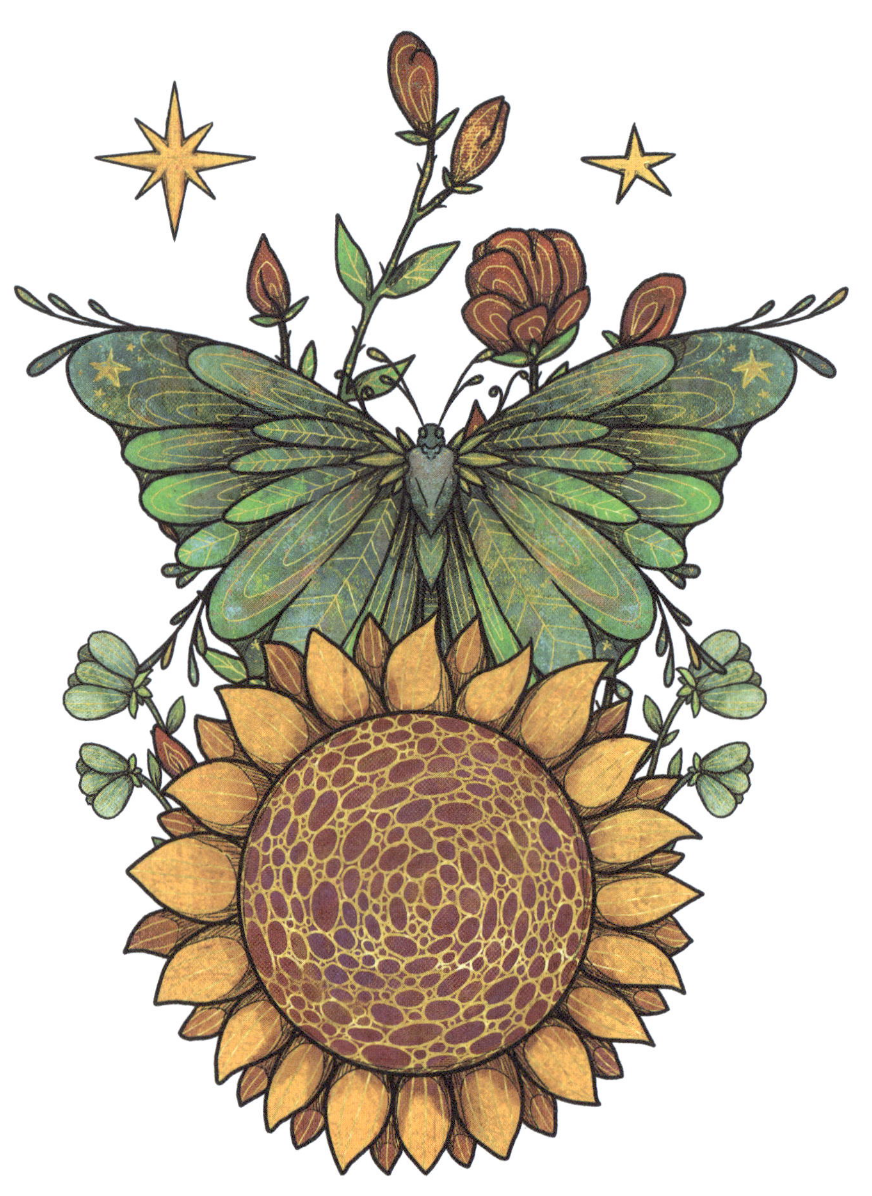

# Introduction

The wheel of the year turns and seasons shift, a dancing pattern of life, death, and transformation, weaving together all that was, is, and shall be. Each of us is woven into the year's turning, bodies of land sustained by the same earth, air, fire, and water that sustained our ancestors and will sustain all who come after us. All of us are shaped by and shape our entanglements—the well-being of the land, our bodies, and our communities intimately interconnected through a deep kinship. And even though we might forget our interconnectedness, the land always remembers.

*The Apothecary of Belonging* is an invitation back into the wisdom that, by being of the land, we have always belonged. While many of us may feel disconnected from the land and one another, through working with the seasons of the year we can partake in a profound reconciliation of all parts of ourselves back home to the land, our bodies, and our communities. Within these pages, we'll work with plant allies and simple rituals to connect with the energy of each season, mixing practical herbalism with inner work, mapping pathways of wisdom, well-being, and sacred relationships.

While this is a book mostly about the seasons of the lands we live with, in many ways it is also a book about bodies. For we are all land—*there is no other*—and though we may call land by many names, it is from a body of land that we are formed and it is as a body of land that we experience life. We are our physical bodies, mental bodies, emotional heart bodies, and bodies that are shrines for our infinite spirit. We are bodies of land, sea, and sky, as well as bodies that hold memories and stories experienced in our present life, inherited from our family and cultural lines, and carried for generations yet to be. As we seek out belonging and the places in the land within and around us in most need of healing, we travel through time, to sites of old pain and early wounds in the past, all while uprooting the belief that healing is an act of individual willpower and moving forward into futures that we are pulling toward us as much as we are being pulled toward them. Exploring seasonal rhythms of kinship helps us recognize what it is we want to make time and space for, developing the ability to cultivate connection in our lives no matter where we come from or where we might be going.

There are so many ways our ability to *feel* our belonging can be disrupted. Many of us have complex direct or ancestral experiences of displacement, migration, settlement, and return. Or we have challenging experiences with our family of origin or cultural upbringing that have made us feel like an "other" from an early age. Pernicious and overt systems of oppression work to divide up land—including our land-bodies—keeping us separated by fear-based borders and creating uncertainty around our own inherent dignity and sacredness. What I hope to explore with you in *The Apothecary of Belonging* is how, rather than a hindrance, the complexity of our land-bodies is an affirmation of our belonging to one another. We are already kin, but it takes practice to develop an intentional and healing relationship with the land and one another.

While the tools needed to dismantle oppressive systems will be as diverse as the people, places, and creatures living under them, there are some simple and useful earth-centered practices everyone can engage with. The central practice I hope to offer is finding connection with the seasonal rhythms of the land as a process of coming home to the healing seasons of your body and the kinship of community. When we begin our healing work from a place of deep knowing we already belong—being inherently of the land—we can begin to untangle beliefs about not being enough, worries about whether we'll ever fit in, or concerns about finding a place for who we are presently as well as who we are becoming. I want you to be guided by the simplicity and complexity of the changing land to accept that you have always belonged and there is abundant space for all of who you are.

Like many of you, I've experienced the discomfort, pain, and confusion of not knowing quite where I belong. As a third-culture kid, mixed womxn, lesbian who is allergic to binaries of all kinds, and someone who has experienced life at different class levels, I've had my share of experiences of believing or being told I don't belong. At the same time, I've had profound experiences of belonging that have been life-changing and hope-sustaining. These experiences of otherness and belonging have shaped my practice as an herbalist, and I'm called to help folks cultivate a resilient and persistent sense of belonging regardless of what culture or family or systems of power may want them to believe is possible.

I can't resolve complicated family stories or identities for you, undo the pain of traumatic experiences, or directly place you in a community of loving peers (*that would be the most amazing superpower!*), but I can help you develop the skills of discernment and self-knowing to recognize how deeply, how profoundly, how beautifully you already belong and how to (re)connect with yourself and the world around you from that place of belonging.

## The Path Ahead

Within *The Apothecary of Belonging* we'll explore with our plant allies how to know ourselves as land and as beings who deeply belong to the land and each other through three primary practices:

- Connecting with and telling the story of the land within us
- Observing and engaging with the seasons of the land around us
- Embodying our kinship through ritual and community practice with the land between us

We'll begin by getting to know our plant allies, our guides to the land around, within, and between us. Then we'll learn about the energetic foundations of traditional western herbalism that flow through the seasons within and around us, exploring ways we can map our inner landscape, and then journey through each of the four seasons with plant allies as our guides and companions. In each seasonal chapter, we'll explore the common themes each part of the year brings as well as ways to connect through your body with the land from breathwork to sacred inquiry.

Each seasonal section also contains an indications-based guide to plant allies for common ailments. Indications are a succinct way of identifying what plants might be most appropriate for a condition through observations of the body. Being able to discern in our body, for example, a dry and hacking cough versus a damp and weak cough is one way to find the best herbs to work with. I have focused on herbs that are generally considered safe with few contraindications, but you should always reference the contraindications appendix as well as look up any plants you want to work with in your trusted *materia medica* or with an herbalist.

You'll also find community clinic suggestions in each seasonal chapter. While not every one of us will or wants to work in a community clinic setting, these ideas can easily be applied to personal apothecaries, households, and friend groups, acting as a guide for sharing herbal gifts and making seasonal donations to herbal calls to action, neighbors, and communities in need. There are also simple tea recipes to support your energy season to season, rituals that can be adapted for solo or community practice, including divination techniques for the inner landscape maps you'll be creating, and lunar blessings to support your remedy-making throughout the year.

## Shared Language

As we journey together, I want to begin by defining some of the terms you'll find here. I use *body* and *land-body* interchangeably to refer not only to the physical body, but our emotional, mental, and energetic bodies as well. When I write of bodies, whether our own individual and finite physical forms or bodies of land, I am speaking of bodies in their most expansive and complex forms.

When I speak of *ancestors*, I am referring to ancestry in the broadest way possible, from familial, cultural, and spiritual ancestors to nonhuman ancestors, including ancestors of place, plant, stone, and water. I use the term *kin* to refer to human and nonhuman kin alike, and sometimes I use terms like *beyond-human kin* and *kindred* to refer to these connections as well. When I write of relationships, it is about relationships of all varieties, not just romantic or family-based. Writing about consultations and clients can refer to professional practice but also encompasses the casual conversations you might have with friends or family members when suggesting herbal care.

Finally, the term *traditional western herbalism* is an imperfect way of describing not only my training and background as an herbalist, but the vast, complicated, and beautiful path of herbalism that such a phrase is trying to encompass. *Traditional* refers to the fact that what I practice is derived from ancient and modern herbal practices, from the evidence-based (including Indigenous science) to the folkloric and magickal. *Western* is much less useful, and I wish there was an alternative for it. Traditional western herbalism has ancient roots in North African, Greek, and Arabic medicine, having journeyed throughout Europe and on to North America, changing and adapting through the centuries. The more I learn about the ways traditional western herbalism developed, the more I've come to appreciate and love its multicultural roots. Terms like *western*, *eastern*, *global south*, and *global north* flatten culture and create misleading binaries about diverse swaths of people, places, and societies. I am sure a better term for this path of herbalism will emerge as language continues to grow more expansive and inclusive. In the meantime, traditional western herbalism is a widely used and recognized umbrella term and a meaningful differentiator from other herbal traditions.

While I'll be wandering through the energetics of traditional western herbalism as a useful form of observation and storytelling, the primary focus of the herbal practice within these pages is building a relationship with our plant allies, which we'll explore in the next chapter.

As we journey along the path of *The Apothecary of Belonging*, may each chapter serve as a map, marked with the places where we might find benevolent plant allies and words of magick, simple rituals and skills of connection, as we trust in our shared belonging and travel the wheel of the year back home together.

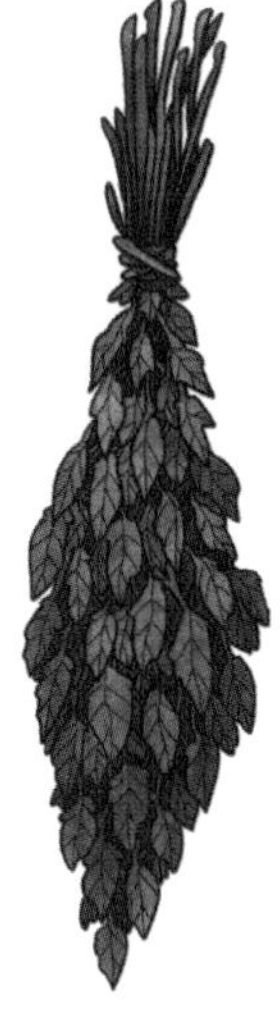

# The Spirits of the Land

## Working with Plant Allies

As an herbalist who works with people and plants for a living and a witch whose path to magick was through the green world, the ways that I know best to help folks find their paths of belonging is through kinship with our plant allies and the land. Throughout *The Apothecary of Belonging* we'll work with plant allies to connect with the energy of the seasons around and within us. Let's begin by exploring what a plant ally is, why it is a useful concept in herbalism, and how it applies to our healing work.

A plant ally is a plant, tree, herb, fungus, alga, or other member of the green world we are in a sacred reciprocal relationship with, helping us to cultivate experiences of well-being in our life. In the sequence of evolution, plants are our elders, having already been present when humans first emerged and witnessing our development throughout millennia. Many plants have evolved alongside us, providing food, shelter, clothing, and medicine. As a species, we have spread their seeds through generations of nomadic and seminomadic life as well as more recently settled and agricultural ways.

Part of my work is to facilitate connections between plants and people. Plant allies can appear to us during times of acute or chronic healing needs. Sometimes plant allies are familiar friends from our younger life such as herbs we grew up with or featured prominently in family meals, while other plant allies may be completely new to us. Often there is an ancestral, spiritual, or cultural connection that becomes obvious once we meet a plant ally, but not always. Some plant allies appear to us in dreams; others show up in the food we are cooking or a childhood memory. Still others appear as gifts, whether from human friends or dropped onto our path by an animal. Plant allies are often eager to show up for us, and we are usually the ones who must practice showing up for them.

The purpose of a plant ally is specific to your relationship with them. Many times plant allies provide relief from suffering, such as chronic pain, heartbreak, or the long recovery from a difficult illness. Usually plant allies come because we have called them, whether consciously or not, and we've been fortunate enough to open up to their help. Some relationships with plant allies last for many years—or a lifetime—but sometimes an ally is here for a season or specific situation and then moves on. Being in relationship with a plant ally often results in growing into your own understanding of who you are and your interconnectedness with the cycles of life, death, and renewal. In other words, plant allies are incredible guardians at the crossroads, helping us move among all parts of our lives, relationships, and communities with greater ease.

When I enter into a relationship with a plant ally (or sometimes wake up to realize that I've been in one without even realizing it—this happens more often than you think!), I try to spend time with the plant in person, from the uncultivated to cultivated spaces where it grows. I try to get to know my plant friend in as many ways and forms as possible, including what time of year they are most abundant, the types of remedies they are used in, and so on, listening with my whole self to their messages, opening up to them as we navigate ways of feeling well together. If I can, I like to carry some of the herb with me, tucked into a small bundle I can wear on my body, connecting me with the very old human practice of wearing plants for various healing and magickal purposes.

Plant allies are incredible facilitators of bonding with the land around and within us, as they are able to travel among memory, dream, and waking consciousness with ease, helping us find what may have been lost along the way. We can incorporate plant allies into our personal practices or honor the connection a client may have with one by incorporating it in appropriate ways in our recommendations. Working with plants of our ancestral or cultural heritage, or helping our clients connect with these types of plants, can be an incredible opportunity for exploring complicated inheritances as well as intergenerational joy.

Finding a plant ally to work with can be as simple as choosing an herb that calls to you and starting there. Sometimes it can be helpful to think about the plants that led you to your interest in herbalism. Other times a plant from your childhood might be the one to speak to you. Let your curiosity guide you and trust the process of knowing yourself better through relationship with your plant allies.

## In Relationship

One of the most important aspects of working with plant allies is how you build a relationship with them. Relationship-building with plants is a combination of both the mundane and magickal—just as it is for most significant relationships in our lives. On the mundane and practical level, consistency (e.g., drinking your tea every day) and observation (e.g., paying attention to the experiences in your body while using the herb) are two very useful tools. Then there are the more magickal and intangible aspects of building a relationship, from choosing to work with a plant ally in a meditation or ritual practice to the ways you might meet in dreams or the sudden insights and body-felt intuitions that come about through the exchange of energy.

On a practical level, as you learn about what herbs might best support your healing needs, I encourage you to start with a few (no more than three at a time), taken singly before moving on to combinations. Working with individual herbs instead of blends at the beginning can help us understand how they show up in the body and interact with our energy systems. Blends can be incorporated later, but it's helpful and informative to start with *simples* (single herbs).

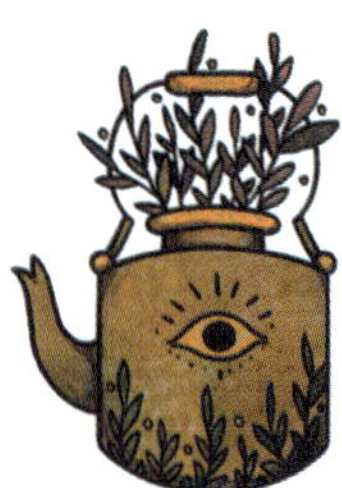

Some of you might be skeptical of or worried about your ability to feel a connection with a plant—it might seem unlikely, if not impossible. It's not unusual for folks to have created a distance between themselves and what they feel in their body as a means of self-protection and survival. The gift of working with plant allies is that they can open the pathways back into the wisdom of our bodies. Plant allies also have a wonderful way of closing the gap between us and the communities we most easily find kinship within, working along invisible pathways between lands to draw us together.

A good place to start in your relationship with a plant ally, besides being curious and showing up to your curiosity, is to ask questions like these:

*Why do I want to work with plants as part of my healing journey?*

*How have I interacted with plants—in medicinal ways or not—in the past?*

*What plants do I currently work with on a regular basis? (Be sure to think about herbs you cook with, the Oats in your oat milk, the Dandelions you see growing up through the cracks in the concrete as you walk to the corner shop, etc.)*

*What are the ways I feel I am in relationship with the plant world? Or do I feel a lack of relationship with the plant world?*

*As I envision a kinship with the plant world, what would that look like for me? What would it feel like?*

We can connect with our plant allies through a variety of simple practices, from learning a plant's folklore, medicinal, and magickal uses; meditating and practicing breathwork with our plant ally; and creating art of our plant, including making your own plant profile filled with your experiences and insights.

## A Simple Plant Ally Ritual

The following ritual outline can be adapted to your needs, including as a community ritual to make a collective remedy or conduct divination for a community query:

- Approach a plant with reverence and openhearted observation.
- Introduce yourself to the plant using names that you were given and/or chose for yourself.
- Offer water, song, or other biodegradable items as an act of gratitude. After asking and whole-body listening for an affirmation, touch the plant and observe its texture, weight, scent, colors, and so on.
- Spend time in a cycle of breath with the plant, imagining your every outbreath becoming their inbreath and vice versa.



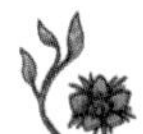

- If you like, practice your favorite form of divination to open lines of communication between you and your plant ally.
- If you are planning on harvesting some of the plants, make a request, telling them what kind of remedy you hope to create with them. Once you have asked and received an affirmation, harvest only an appropriate amount, following earth-centered wildcrafting or harvesting guidelines.
- Make another offering after breathwork, divination, and/or harvesting, and give thanks to the plant and the land for their generosity.


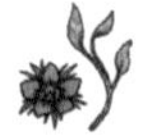

# An Earth-Centered Practice

## Herbal Energetics & Reading the Land

While I trained in traditional western herbalism, I describe my herbal practice as intersectional, approaching those I serve and the plants I work with from a place of compassionate curiosity and embodied wisdom. My practice is earth-centered, recognizing plants themselves as some of our most profound teachers and centering earth-affirming and sustainable choices. I believe herbalists and plant folk should be living resources of herbal tradition and community connectors, and I hope people interacting with my work are reminded that healing is a multifaceted exchange of knowledge from the deeply practical to the intangible, all leading us back to the wisdom that none of us were ever meant to heal alone.

In helping you find a sustainable and enduring practice, I want to share with you the energetic system of traditional western herbalism I work with season to season. Understanding energetics—not only our own personal energy needs and systems, but the energetics of plants—can be one way we transmute knowledge (e.g., what a plant does on a physiological level) into wisdom (e.g., how we best work with a plant for our individual needs and create a relationship with them).

I have found the language of herbal energetics provides a wonderful way to be able to observe, describe, and share stories about our inner experiences. The herbal energetics of traditional western herbalism are just one form of an energetic system, and I hope that if you are reconnecting to herbal traditions of your cultural or spiritual heritage, you also explore the herbal energetics of your ancestral lines.

### Defining Herbal Energetics

The phrase *herbal energetics* gets used in a number of ways, including as an interchangeable term for herbal actions (i.e., astringent, digestive, emollient, etc.), but energetics are a separate form of nonmedical terminology arising from a time when physical observation was the primary tool of diagnosis.

Herbal energetics developed from using the elements to define the qualities of plants, diseases, and people, codifying the physical observations relied on by practitioners of ancient Egyptian, Greek, and Arabic traditions (i.e., the foundational cultural traditions of traditional western herbalism that made their way between Europe, Southwest Asia, North Africa, and eventually North America). The core of the energetic system of traditional western herbalism is the four elements of earth, air, fire, and water, laying the foundation for concepts like humoral theory, a variety of esoteric and astrological principles, and the six tissue states. Elemental systems are varied even within traditional western herbalism, shaped by the people practicing them and changing between practitioners and generations. Even the ancient Greeks, who laid significant groundwork for elemental practice contradicted themselves and each other when defining the elements, and we should all feel free to keep adapting, reconsidering, and adding to them.

In addition to the vast lineage of traditional western herbalism, my magickal training and practice as a modern Pagan and Witch, ancestral and Indigenous traditions, and direct experience shape my understanding of the elements, too. It is important when studying any modality to seek out what works for us, engage with but not become hindered by what challenges us, and ultimately choose the path most relevant, least harmful, and most inspiring to us and the land, people, and nonhuman kin we serve.

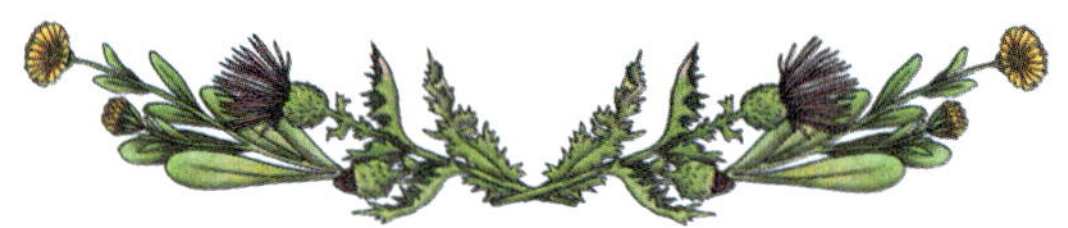

## Four Elements

Let's start with defining the four elements, which will help us understand the six tissue states we'll be exploring next. In the Greek tradition (most likely influenced by older Egyptian practice) the four elements are categorized by the primary qualities of heat, cold, dryness, and damp as follows:

Fire is Hot & Dry
Air is Hot & Damp
Earth is Cold & Dry
Water is Cold & Damp

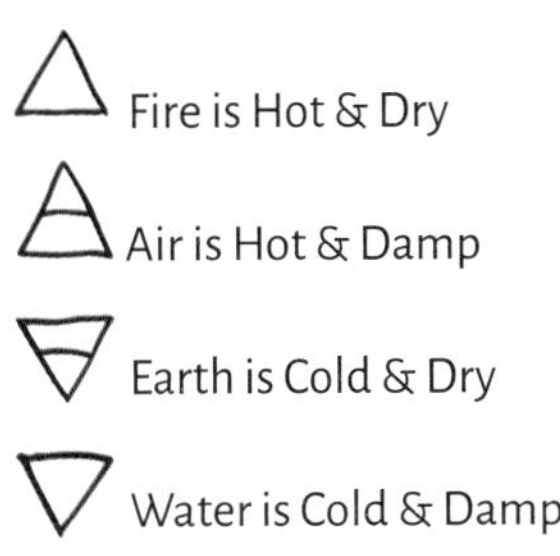

The four elements were further defined by secondary qualities we could consider their actions or tones, moving from heavy to light:

- **Earth:** Heavy, firm, stable, dense, sustained and enduring energy that centers and moves downward
- **Water:** Moderate heaviness, soft, slippery, smooth; easily adapts to different shapes and spaces, receptive
- **Air:** Light, thin, subtle, adaptable, porous, warm; moves energy upward
- **Fire:** Absolute lightness, bright, very rare; transforms and transmutes energy into other qualities

To understand these elemental qualities we have to do a bit of "yes, and" thinking. Yes, fire is literally hot in temperature *and* the quality of hot also describes the heat of life. Within traditional western herbalism the vital spirits giving life to the body (also known as *pneuma* and similar in nature to descriptions of *prana* in Ayurveda or *chi* in Traditional Chinese Medicine) were understood by ancient Greek physicians as warm and radiating life-giving breath. So, hot describes the heat of life in contrast to the coldness of death. The element of air possesses less hot energy than fire but is seen as carrying the warm breath of life throughout the body. In modern western herbalism we would describe many air herbs as circulatory tonics delivering nutrients and warmth, as well as strengthening the heart (a seat of *pneuma* and heat in the body).

One way to start connecting to the somatic experience of the four elements in your body is to describe your sensory experiences with elemental language. A pain in your back may feel hot and burning; feelings of contentment might seem earthy and grounded; a period of sadness might feel like you're treading water;

or the cough you have makes it feel like you can't fully fill your lungs with air. We can also connect with the elements of plants (e.g., the mucilaginous, watery nature of *emollient herbs*) and diseases (e.g., the hot fire energy of a fever).

In addition to becoming aware of the elemental language we already use, we can begin to observe elemental energy in the four seasons. The elements correspond to seasons in traditional western herbalism as

- Spring: Air
- Summer: Fire
- Autumn: Earth
- Winter: Water

While every season carries with it the energy of all four elements, our ancient herbal ancestors observed that certain elemental energies were more pronounced at different times of year. I encourage you to pay attention to the abundance or lack of elemental energies where you live, from the intensity of water during monsoon seasons or the strength of the air as wind coming down from the mountains during spring. Throughout the seasonal chapters we'll explore the connections between the elemental energies of the land around us and our own inner landscape.

### *Air*

- Too much air can lead to overstimulation, mental fatigue, anxiety, panic, and the Tension tissue state.
- Too little air can create brain fog, restlessness, poor executive functioning, lack of vision, and the Relaxation and/or Stagnation tissue state.
- A balance of air supports intellectual capacity and problem-solving, the ability to communicate authentically, and a balanced cerebral state.

### *Fire*

- Too much fire can lead to irritation, inflammation, anger, burnout, and the Heat and/or Tension tissue states.


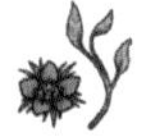

- Too little fire can lead to poor digestion, lack of inspiration, lack of hope, and the Cold, Stagnation, and/or Relaxation tissue states.
- A balance of fire helps us move energy, digest and assimilate nutrients, and support our inherent vitality.

## *Water*

- Too much water can lead to retention of fluids and feelings, difficulty setting boundaries, addictive habits, and the Cold, Relaxation, and/or Stagnation tissue states.
- Too little water can create lack of empathy and flexibility as well as a difficulty connecting, and the Dryness, Heat, and/or Tension tissue states.
- A balance of water supports emotional intelligence, empathy, healthy fluids in the body, and expanded states of perception of ourselves and our world.

## *Earth*

- Too much earth can lead to stagnation, slow digestion, lethargy, overwork, cynicism, and the Cold, Relaxation, and/or Stagnation tissue states.
- Too little earth can lead to lack of stamina, poor absorption of nutrients, difficulty being present in the body, and the Heat and/or Dry tissue states.
- A balance of earth supports embodiment, sovereignty of self and security of identity, and a resilient physical form.

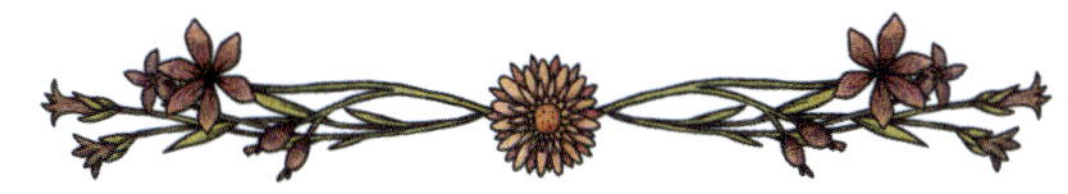

## None of Us Perfect, All of Us Whole

Having worked with the four sacred elements for a few decades, I love how the system is both simple and accessible while allowing for endless complexity. Each of us is born whole and holy and with certain elemental dispositions. Some of us are fierier and quicker to act; others are slower, steadier, and more considered in our actions. Some of us have an ocean's depth capacity to feel; others carry an endless line of energy for studying and philosophizing.

Each of us has all four elements within us, and we journey through life developing, forgetting, and learning anew what it is to feel settled in the land within and around us. The abundance of water one person carries nurtures the spaces within another who is learning to flow with the tide of their feelings. A friend's earthiness supports the longevity of another's airy visions. We come to know ourselves and our world by seeking out connections, allowing ourselves to be found, and expanding our perceptions of ourselves, our communities, and our world. Within the framework of traditional western herbalism we come to know ourselves, in part, by finding ways to support the elemental energy we have in abundance and seeking out ways to enrich the areas of our elemental self needing extra support.

## Six Tissue States

Building on the foundation of the four elements, the more recently developed tissue states act as observational tools to describe the qualities of diseases and discomforts, as well as the landscape of our bodies and the ways that plant medicine affects that landscape. Folks familiar with other systems of herbal energetics will find similarities between the tissue states and the doshas of Ayurvedic tradition, the five elements of Traditional Chinese Medicine, and so on.

Throughout this book, I refer to the tissue states in terms friendliest to modern ears, but I also want to highlight that each tissue state has many names. Let's look at these for each tissue state so you'll be able to navigate your way through historical and modern documents on this interesting part of traditional western herbalism with a little more ease:

- **Heat:** Hot, Irritation, Excitation, Irritation, Choleric, Vasoexaggeration



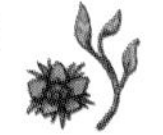

- **Cold:** Depression, Melancholic, Vasodepression
- **Tension:** Wind, Constriction, Vasoconstriction
- **Relaxation:** Lax, Atony, Dilation, Vasodilation
- **Dryness:** Dry, Atrophic, Sanguine, Vasotrophesy
- **Stagnation:** Damp, Torpor, Torpid, Vasoatony

At their core, the tissue states are simply ways of describing the four elements and their actions in our bodies, in plants, and through diseases and discomforts.

- Heat describes the presence of fire.
- Cold describes the presence of earth.
- Tension describes the presence of air.
- Relaxation describes the presence of water.
- Dryness describes the presence of fire and air.
- Stagnation describes the presence of earth and water.

Drawing on their elemental nature, the tissue states bring additional insight in describing temperature (Hot or Cold), moisture (Dry or Damp), and tone (Tense or Relaxed). People tend to have an inherent baseline of tissue states (e.g., someone who runs hot all the time versus someone who is always cold); diseases or discomforts have tissue states (e.g., a fever is a condition of excess Heat); and plants have tissue states (e.g., *Avena sativa* carries the energy of the Relaxed tissue state). In practice, if I observe excess Heat and Tension in a client, say from a headache that makes them feel overheated, I will probably turn to Cold (e.g., anti-inflammatories) and Relaxing (gentle sedatives) remedies to help them.

While tissue states are not diagnostic, when they are combined with tools like evidence-based *materia medica*, they serve as a helpful compass, directing us toward what plants might be appropriate for an issue among the vast catalog available. Throughout the seasonal chapters I'll refer to the tissue states as a way to connect with the energies of each season as well as part of the indications-based apothecary recommendations.

What follows are summaries of each of the six tissue states, focusing on how they affect our energy and our bodies, including body system function. I point out the types of herbs that embody the energy of each as well as the gifts of each tissue state since we need all of them to live. In the recommendations for alleviating imbalances brought on by a tissue state, I list my favorite plant ally to balance that state first, but you'll find plenty of plant allies to connect with in each list. Many herbs are listed for multiple tissue states because our plant allies are incredibly adaptable, possessing a multitude of healing gifts and acting multidirectionally when it comes to balancing out energy systems.

You'll also find key phrases for each imbalanced tissue state. One of the best ways to understand tissue states is through connecting with these expressions of the elements in our personal experience. I encourage you to say each phrase out loud, taking note of which ones resonate with you. Discovering your inherent tissue states—such as whether you're more prone to overheating or are always cold—can be a great way of understanding and finding language for your energy and how it expresses itself.

### *Heat*

Heat is a state of overstimulation where energy has tipped toward overactive. Organs seem to be working too quickly but do not perform their functions well or sustainably; illnesses and discomfort generate heat from fevers to inflammation. Heat herbs are spicy, produce sweating, and are energizing in nature. The gifts of Heat are life, energy, and intuition. Signs of excess Heat include hyper-conditions—hypersensitive, overstimulated, angry, agitated, irritated, and inflamed.

**Heat Key Phrases**

*I'm angry.*

*I find everything agitating/irritating.*

*I'm nervous/anxious all the time.*

*I'm bored.*

*I see red.*

*Anger is the quickest way to get people to pay attention when I'm overwhelmed.*



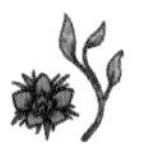

*I don't feel powerful.*

*I want everyone to know how powerful I am.*

**Plant Allies:** Cooling herbs, sedatives, and bitters. Lemon Balm (*Melissa officinalis*), Ashwagandha (*Withania somnifera*), Chamomile (*Matricaria chamomilla*), Dandelion (*Taraxacum officinale*), Elder (*Sambucus nigra*), Lavender (*Lavandula* spp.), Passionflower (*Passiflora incarnata*), Rose (*Rosa* spp.), Skullcap (*Scutellaria lateriflora*), Vervain (*Verbena officinalis, V. hastata*).

## Cold

The Cold tissue state is the *hypo-* to the *hyper-* of the Heat tissue state. Everything is understimulated, including the body's vital energy and ability to maintain a healthy cellular habitat. With excess Cold the efficiency of functions is greatly decreased, leading to a sluggishness in body systems. Cold herbs are sedating and cooling, and help to preserve moisture. The gifts of Cold are boundaries, stillness, and longevity. Signs of excess Cold include hypo-conditions, poor circulation, brain fog, slow digestion, and poor absorption of nutrients.

**Cold Key Phrases**

*I am sad.*

*I'm unsatisfied.*

*I feel like I'm treading water or fighting to stay afloat.*

*I don't feel connected to anything.*

*I lack inspiration and energy.*

*I feel the weariness in my bones.*

*I'm tired all of the time.*

*I can't get warm.*

**Plant Allies:** Warming, spicy, aromatic, and stimulating herbs. Holy Basil (*Ocimum tenuiflorum*), Ashwagandha (*Withania somnifera*), Dandelion (*Taraxacum officinale*), Gotu Kola (*Centella asiatica*), Lemon Balm (*Melissa officinalis*) when combined with warming herbs, Milky Oat (*Avena sativa*), Rhodiola (*Rhodiola rosea*), Rose (*Rosa* spp.), St. Joan's Wort (*Hypericum perforatum*).

## *Tension*

The Tension tissue state has a very "this-or-that" nature to it, resulting in feeling there is little room for nuance energetically or physically when out of balance. Excess Tension can lead to body systems running too under- or overstimulated and energy feeling like it is *on* all the time until it suddenly is not. Tension herbs are astringent and toning, helping to regulate body systems. The gifts of Tension are communication, focus, and observation. Signs of excess Tension include insomnia, irritability, restlessness, muscle spasms and cramping, burnout, and mood swings.

**Tension Key Phrases**

*I am so stressed out.*

*I can't relax.*

*There's never enough time.*

*I'm feeling squeezed/tight/restricted.*

*I feel sharp/on edge/anxious.*

*My stomach is in knots.*

*Everyone is dancing on my last nerve!*

*I don't even know where to start about how I'm feeling.*

**Plant Allies:** Relaxants, adaptogens, and acrid herbs. Milky Oat (*Avena sativa*), Ashwagandha (*Withania somnifera*), Chamomile (*Matricaria chamomilla*), Eleuthero (*Eleutherococcus senticosus*), Lavender (*Lavandula* spp.), Passionflower (*Passiflora incarnata*), Reishi (*Ganoderma lucidum*), Skullcap (*Scutellaria lateriflora*), Vervain (*Verbena officinalis, V. hastata*).

## *Relaxation*

The prominent feature of the Relaxation tissue state is a lack of tone, leading to collapse and overflow. Excess Relaxation can bring on conditions such as


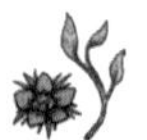

low-level but chronic fatigue as well as water retention as the body struggles to process fluids, nutrients, and feelings. Relaxation herbs are calming and deeply relaxing, alleviating emotional and physical tension. The gifts of Relaxation are peace and adaptability. Signs of excess Relaxation include leaky conditions such as a runny nose, diarrhea, excess mucus, and heavy menstruation, as well as lack of energy and mental clarity.

**Relaxation Key Phrases**

*I don't know how to share/put into words what I'm feeling.*

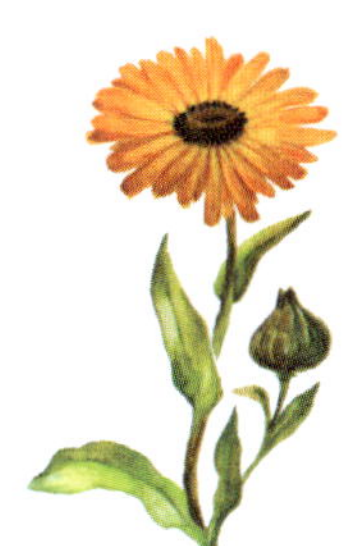

*I feel hopeless.*

*Getting up in the mornings is the worst.*

*Everything is a struggle.*

*I can't take the pressure.*

*I don't know where my edges are.*

*I feel drained.*

*I can't tell the difference between my feelings and the feelings of others.*

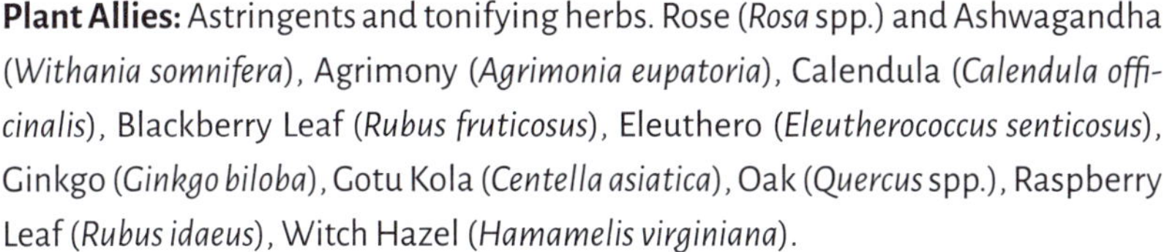

**Plant Allies:** Astringents and tonifying herbs. Rose (*Rosa* spp.) and Ashwagandha (*Withania somnifera*), Agrimony (*Agrimonia eupatoria*), Calendula (*Calendula officinalis*), Blackberry Leaf (*Rubus fruticosus*), Eleuthero (*Eleutherococcus senticosus*), Ginkgo (*Ginkgo biloba*), Gotu Kola (*Centella asiatica*), Oak (*Quercus* spp.), Raspberry Leaf (*Rubus idaeus*), Witch Hazel (*Hamamelis virginiana*).

## Dryness

The Dryness tissue state arises from lack of moisture in the body leading to brittleness, inflexibility, and stiffness. Excess Dryness can lead to exhaustion from undernourishment and difficulty in the body's regenerative functions. Dryness herbs are stimulating and energizing, restoring strength and toning body systems. The gifts of Dryness are clarification and inspiration. Signs of excess Dryness include long and tedious recovery from illness, dry and/or flaking skin, brittle hair and nails, low endurance, and irregular fluids, including menstruation and urination.

**Dryness Key Phrases**

*I can't focus (meditate, sit still, etc.).*

*I want to run away.*

*I feel like I catch every cold that comes my way.*

*I'm all over the place.*

*I just don't feel like myself.*

*I've used up all my resources.*

*I feel depleted.*

*I feel that no matter what I do, nothing helps.*

**Plant Allies:** Oily, sweet (i.e., adaptogens), and demulcent herbs. Milky Oat (*Avena sativa*), Aloe Vera (*Aloe* spp.), Ashwagandha (*Withania somnifera*), Fenugreek (*Trigonella foenum-graecum*), Gotu Kola (*Centella asiatica*), Licorice (*Glycyrrhiza glabra*), Marshmallow (*Althea officinalis*), Plantain (*Plantago major, P. lanceolata*), Reishi (*Ganoderma lucidum*), Sage (*Salvia officinalis*).

## *Stagnation*

In the Stagnation tissue state fluids collect inside the body as opposed to flowing freely through and out of the body (as in Relaxation). With Stagnation, the ability to move fluids out of the body is impaired—whether through the lack of digestive function or elimination—and the buildup of fluids or energy in one part of the body leads to congestion. Stagnation herbs are moisture-producing, nutrient-building, and adaptogenic. The gifts of Stagnation are manifestation and structure. Signs of excess Stagnation include swelling (including swollen lymph glands), water retention, poor immunity, slow elimination, and low mood and energy.

**Stagnation Key Phrases**

*I don't care.*

*I'm so overwhelmed I've become indifferent.*

*I feel stuck.*


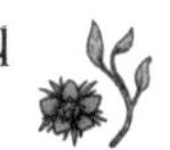

*I feel the weight of the world (compassion fatigue).*

*I feel like I'm drowning/under the surface.*

*I feel bloated and swampy.*

*Everyone seems to know what they're doing except me.*

*My feelings are hurt and I can't move through it.*

**Plant Allies:** Bitters, circulatory and metabolic tonics. Lemon Balm (*Melissa officinalis*), Ashwagandha (*Withania somnifera*), Dandelion (*Taraxacum officinale*), Eleuthero (*Eleutherococcus senticosus*), Ginger (*Zingiber officinale*), Ginkgo (*Ginkgo biloba*), Hawthorn (*Crataegus monogyna*), Hyssop (*Hyssopus officinalis*), Sage (*Salvia officinalis*), St. Joan's Wort (*Hypericum perforatum*), Turmeric (*Curcuma longa*).

## Herbal Energetics in Practice

Over the years, what I've found most useful about tissue states is that the words and concepts not only provide a sensory-rich language to describe people, conditions, and plants, but an easy way to explore healing needs, including medical terminology, in a language more accessible and more easily felt on a somatic level. If you want to incorporate herbal energetics into your practice, I recommend starting by categorizing your favorite plant allies, your most common health complaints, and even the weather of each season by element and tissue states. These simple observations will help you become familiar and comfortable with the language of herbal energetics.

One of the greatest benefits of learning herbal energetics, besides connecting us to a legacy of herbal healing, is having a system of discernment at once simple and clarifying while also able to handle complexity. I hope you enjoy learning about and experimenting with tissue states, add to their indications, incorporate your own phrasing, and participate in the unfolding story of traditional western herbalism—all of us sharing our observations and insights with one another continues to make practices like herbal energetics profoundly useful.

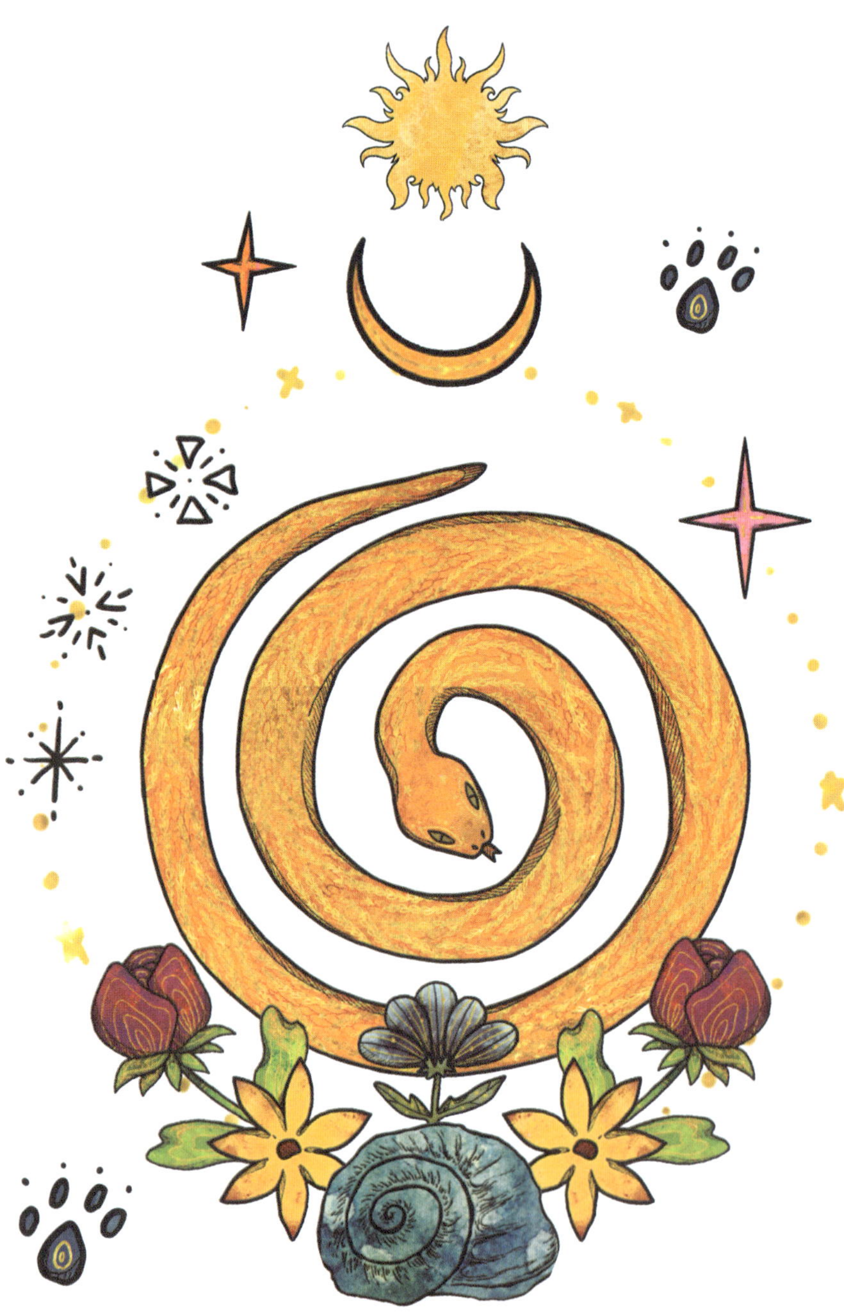

# *Making Our Own Maps*

## Creating an Oracle of Belonging

The human need to be found is an old one, reflected in our prehistoric art of handprints and hunting grounds, ancient maps and celestially aligned megaliths. As we travel together through the seasons, I want to offer you a tool for finding and being found while exploring the land around, between, and within you. An oracle of belonging or oracle map is a physical representation of our inner landscape that helps us recognize the patterns of our stories so we can connect more deeply to who we are, to the land that holds us, and to the communities that know us (whether or not we've met them yet).

I have been creating versions of oracle maps inspired by ancestral and modern traditions of magick since I first learned you could toss rocks or sticks on markings on the ground for divination. Over the years, I've incorporated correspondence systems, astrological wisdom, and deeply personal imagery as a way to understand who I've been, where I am right now, and who I am becoming. Later, when I began seeing herbalism clients, I found oracle maps a useful tool of observation and self-inquiry, helping folks connect with their healing needs and find where they felt most at home in their lives.

What follows is my simple guide to creating your very own oracle of belonging to use as a somatic tool of self-inquiry and gentle divination on your journey throughout the wheel of the year and the many seasons of your life.

### Mapping Our Inner Landscapes

While individual oracle maps will be unique, the underlying structure is one of kinship and correspondence. From astrological maps to megalithic carvings, prehistoric life and myths illustrated on ancient cave walls and humoral charts in medical texts to detailed guides of the upper, middle, and lower worlds painted on drums, I feel deeply connected to our species' impulse for recordkeeping and creating easy-to-share infographics, mnemonic devices, and art. I've long been enamored with the correspondence tables found in old herbals, ancient grimoires, and modern spellbooks alike helping us make sense of the immensity of life by charting the patterns of existence. As we explore belonging together, it feels appropriate to draw on this tradition of synthesizing experience and knowledge into something that can be looked at, held, and used as a tool for storytelling and finding one another.

An oracle of belonging is born from our skills of observation developed through our seasonal practices, acting as a map of our inner landscape and a tool to help us find the words to tell the stories of our experiences. Sharing stories, being heard, and creating connection in the telling and hearing of these personal myths are powerful acts of belonging, carrying us through the year, illuminating our entanglements, and weaving us into the wisdom of the land and our communities. Creating your own oracle of belonging is a way to know the land within you by mapping out your inner landscape on *your own* terms and with *your own* tools. Our oracle maps help us better recognize the land around us while coming to know the land of others, intermingled along the edges of who we are, what we know, and what we don't know.

What I love about the oracle-making process is we get to explore the landscape of our experiences and the legacy of patterns handed down to us through the generations—from star maps, harvest cycles, knitting patterns, language structures, song rhythms, and more—while already being home. We can start to recognize the land of our body from a place of knowing that the land around us has never forgotten us, no matter where migration, settlement, assimilation, conquest, or far-flung diaspora may have taken us or our ancestors. We map our inner landscapes, allowing them to be as complex as we are, changing with our tectonic shifts or gentle seasons, and illuminating our healing needs like constellations.

While modern maps are easy to associate with conquest and dominion, the actual art of mapmaking—delineating features in the landscape, charting seasons, moon cycles, and celestial movements—is an old human practice of connection dating back thousands of years. Working from a place of intersectionality and inclusivity where a map is seen as a library of living stories, an oracle map can become a tool of liberatory healing.


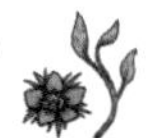

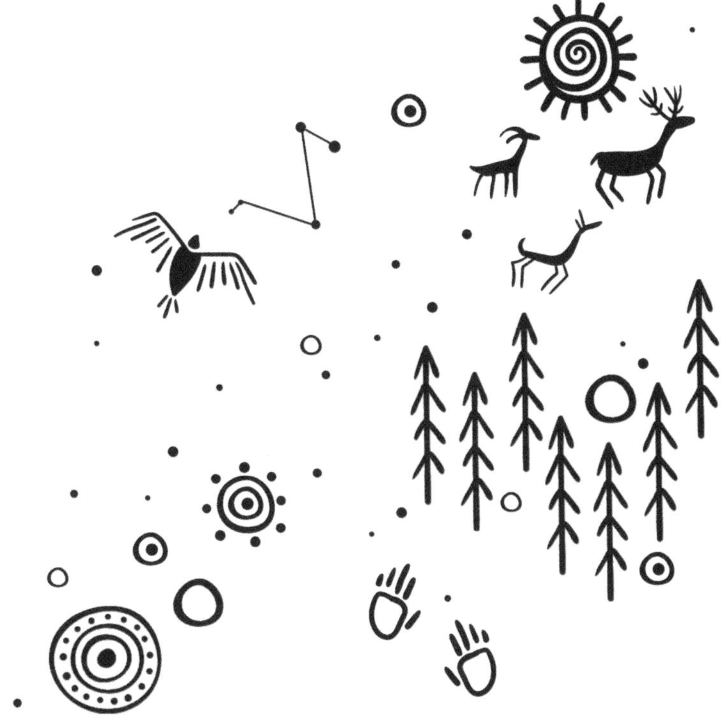

Our oracle maps are a means of navigation, of relationship, and of curiosity. Exploring our inner landscapes and illustrating what we see on our oracle maps are a way to reassess, release, and adjust the landmarks of our life, our identities, and our experiences that were named for us instead of by us. In the same way that places on the land around us are being released from the history of conquest and given old or renewed names centering Indigenous people or honoring modern figures better aligned with the land and its communities, we can begin the processes of rooting out societal expectations and internalized oppressions, forced languages and cultural mandates, and interpersonal beliefs from our internal land-body. We can also explore challenging feelings of shame and guilt that can arise as we reckon with the harmful impact of our species on each other, the land, and our nonhuman kin, exploring the borderlands of our fear and discomfort and how they show up in our inner landscape as felt experiences.

As we create our oracles, we make space for reconnection to the parts of ourselves we want to call home, cultivating restoration and agency as we literally make space for all of who we are. Mapping our inner knowing and resilience reorients us toward our values and our deep well of wisdom, letting us recognize beloved communities while protecting us from the pitfalls of conformity that can lead us away from our most sacred connections. Working with our inner landscape hones our skill of discernment and healing relationships—not because we will be able to attain some sort of infallible wisdom of what is happening for us internally, but because we become better equipped to recognize when something feels off and reorient to pathways that feel honest, good, and appropriate again.

## Divining the Path

When approached as a tool of self-inquiry and divination, our oracle maps help us connect with and name what is happening in our inner landscape, allowing us to map our finite experiences in an infinite universe. Your oracle map can be a tool of exploration, from incorporating it in pathworkings or meditations to exploring the seasonal shifts of your inner landscape through looking at seasonal themes or the sacred inquiry questions you'll encounter in the seasonal apothecaries.

Since an oracle of belonging is a deeply personal tool, it can easily be used with your preferred divination system. Lots (e.g., runes or ogham), charms, seeds, grains, shells, stones, bones, or dice can be tossed on the oracle map. They can be used as a spread for oracle or tarot cards (i.e., cards pulled for different places on the oracle map). Pendulums can be suspended above them, and so on. As we'll explore in the next section, you can place divinatory markers on your oracle map, from astrological glyphs to elemental symbols, that serve as little doorways or placeholders of information and deeper meaning. Throughout this book you'll find examples of oracle map divination, where I've created sample maps to inspire your own creations for your healing practice.

## Creating Your Oracle

The beauty of creating your own oracle of belonging is giving form to your own inner landscape instead of your homeland being drawn by someone else. While all of us are shaped by our relationships, our cultures, the land around us, and our ancestry, the oracle map is where we get to *choose* what we record, illustrate, and name the symbols of our land-body experiences. Practically speaking, your oracle can be made with any medium of your choosing, from a drawing, collage, or painting to a quilt, embroidered, knit, or woven cloth to carved wood or stone, and so on. Your oracle map could be one piece (e.g., a painted cloth) or many pieces (a collection of painted stones or deck of cards). I recommend choosing a medium that speaks to you and working from there, knowing you can always start again or change things up—your oracle map is meant to grow and change with you.

Most importantly, create your oracle of belonging knowing it is not meant to be shared with anyone, except perhaps your closest loved ones. You might even ask yourself when starting to work on your oracle map: *Who am I when no one else is looking? What do I look like when I am being seen in all my wholeness?*

Inspiration for your oracle map might come from these areas:

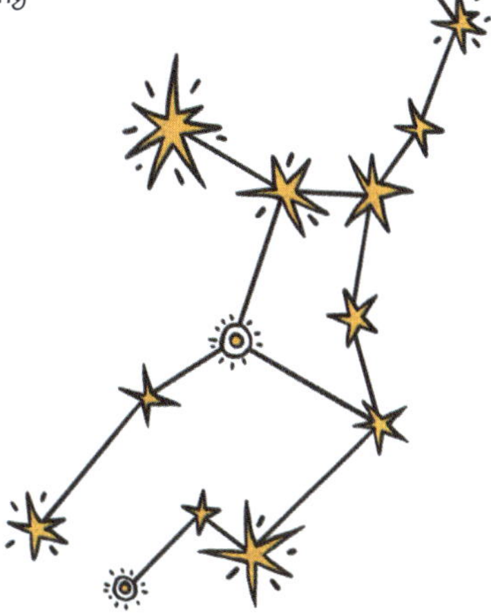

- Megalithic sites and prehistoric art
- Cultural and spiritual imagery, including divinities or holy ones and their symbols
- Fantasy maps from books you love
- Symbols from your favorite systems of divination
- Astrological tradition (e.g., parts or all of your birth chart, planetary glyphs, the zodiac wheel)

- Energy systems such as the cauldrons of poesy, meridian lines, chakras, ley lines, or more from your spiritual and/or cultural practices
- The land you live with, including culturally or personally significant landmarks
- Plant and tree allies

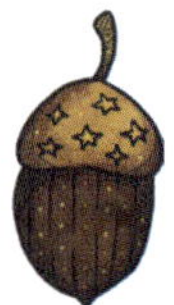 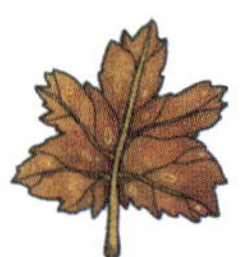 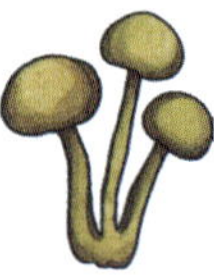

The design of your oracle map can be as simple or complex as you want, from basic geometric symbols to a topographical landscape with geological layers, tidal patterns, and the flyways of birds. You can have different body systems literally or symbolically represented (e.g., a forest for the lungs, rivers for the nervous system, sun and moon for the eyes) as well as the elements and whatever energetic system(s) you use in your practice.

Let yourself dream with your oracle map, imagining ways to bring more of yourself into the world, whether you're reconnecting with ancestral wisdom or expanding out from narrow family, social, or cultural environments. In many ways, creating an oracle map is a healing ritual by naming and calling in ways of being that feel whole and holy. Creating an oracle map, with all of its symbolism and land-centered qualities, can feel more inviting and inspiring than the flat, if accurate and necessary, descriptors of therapeutic care and hoped-for outcomes. While we might know, for example, that we need to increase our mobility through reducing inflammation in our joints and improving circulation, we might feel more able to connect with that healing path by visualizing it on our oracle map as a cool, windswept valley of unhindered movement and you, as a raven, flying through it with ease.

A simple oracle of belonging structure might include the following:

- Representation of the four elements
- Representations of body systems

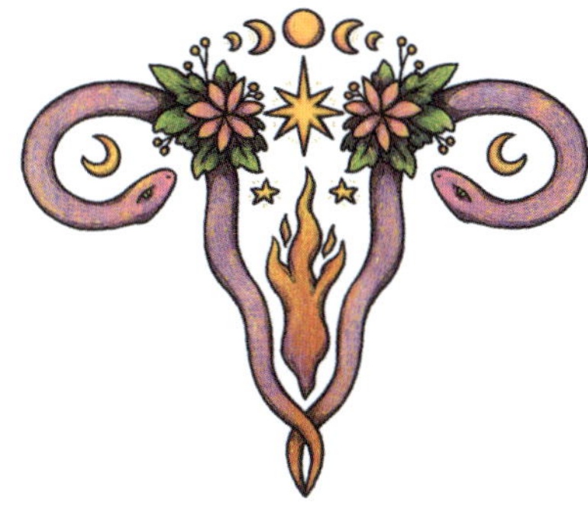

- A place for your ancestors and/or holy ones
- A place for the strange, uncomfortable, and/or unfamiliar (i.e., honoring your shadows)
- A place for what you are hoping to find healing, resolution, or reconnection with
- Markings for significant life experiences

Some of my favorite plant allies for awakening intuition and connecting with the subtle energies of our inner worlds include Mugwort (*Artemisia vulgaris*), Rose (*Rosa* spp.), Yarrow (*Achillea millefolium*), Thyme (*Thymus vulgaris*), and Peppermint (*Mentha piperita*). Once you've created your oracle of belonging, you can bring it to life with a simple elemental blessing by holding it to your body (earth), breathing on it (air), anointing it with your fluid (water), and gazing at it (fire).

## Practical Uses

Beyond our somatic exploration and divination, your oracle map can be used in a number of magickal ways:

- A place to create an altar or as artwork for your altar
- A symbol of you in healing rituals, focusing on the area in most need of healing
- A map for trancework or pathworking

- A place to charge magickal tools, stones, and herbal remedies for your personal healing work
- A useful means of exploring the energetic system of traditional western herbalism as represented by different landscapes (e.g., representing your tendency to run hot and dry with a beautiful high desert landscape, helping you understand how Heat and Dryness act in your body)

You can also make oracle maps of the land you are in kinship with to deepen your connections, of significant relationships that highlight you and the other person(s), and/or you can make community oracle maps.

## The Community Oracle

While an oracle of belonging can be a deeply personal practice, we can also use it as a tool of community connection. Working with any system of healing should draw us through our inner worlds and into stronger connections with our communities. Community oracle maps are interesting guides to the visions, hopes, and spirits embodied by a group and can become especially poignant when a community exists because of some connection to place. By making an oracle map that represents shared space, we can begin to explore the landscape of a community that lies beyond the *work* of a group into the *feeling* of a group. Community oracle maps are constructed in the same way as personal oracle maps, focusing on significant landmarks, pathways of belonging, crossroads of conflict, and ancient woodlands of tradition.

Like personal oracles of belonging, community oracles can be used for inquiry (e.g., *How is the momentum of spring bringing change to our community landscape?*), for divination, and for healing rituals of all kinds.

## Opening the Oracle

Once you've dreamed of, created, and blessed your oracle of belonging, you can use it as you please, making sure to adjust it as needed as you change and grow. In my own practice, I like to "open" or "wake up" my oracle by speaking a charm before I do any work with it, helping to draw my focus and center me for the work ahead.

 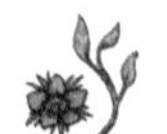 

### *The Oracle of Belonging Blessing*

Adapt the blessing for community practice by changing personal statements to we statements:

*I am listening*
*to my body*
*where I belong*

*to the east and west*
*where I belong*

*to the north and south*
*where I belong*

*between land, sea, and sky*
*where I belong*

*within the embrace of beloved community*
*where I belong*

*I am listening*
*to my body*
*where I belong*

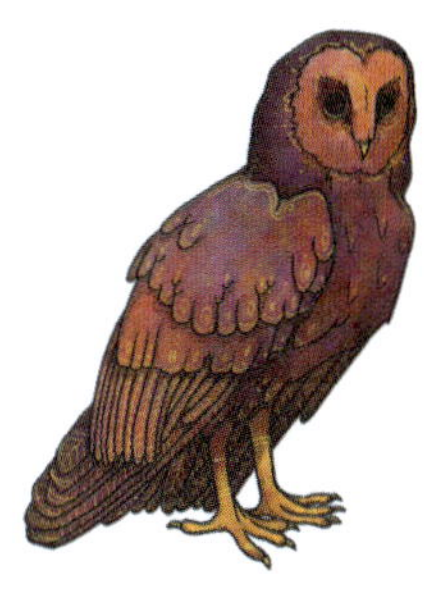

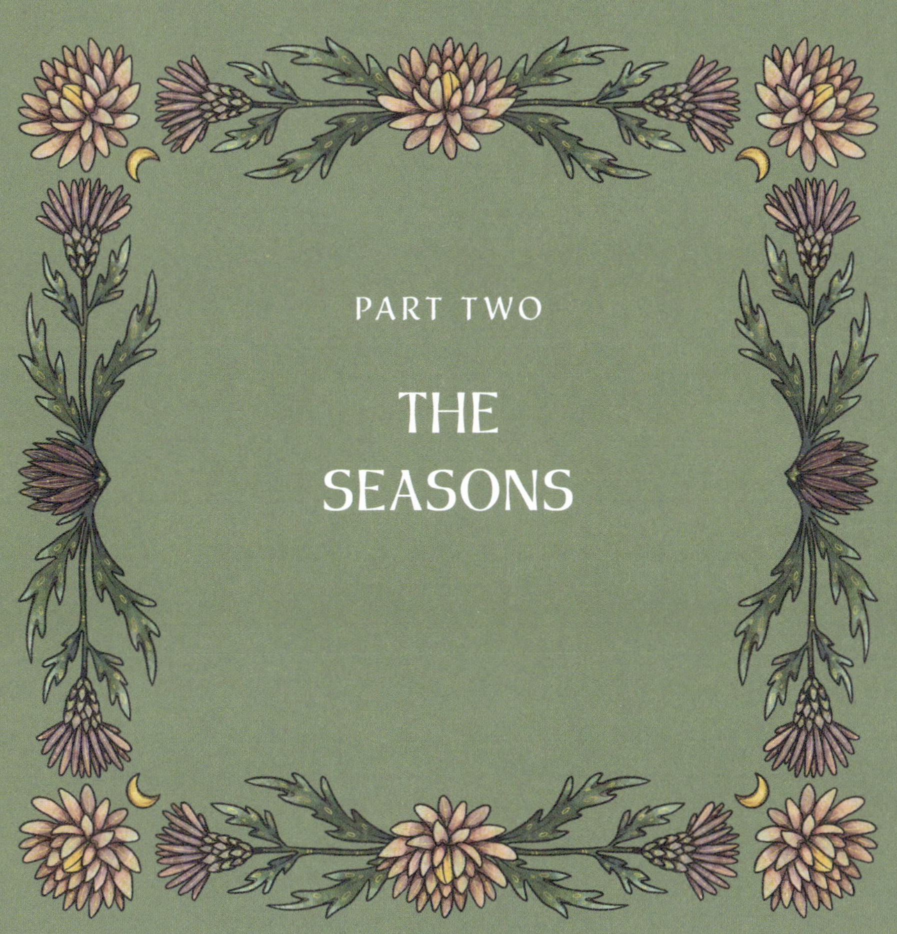

PART TWO

# THE SEASONS

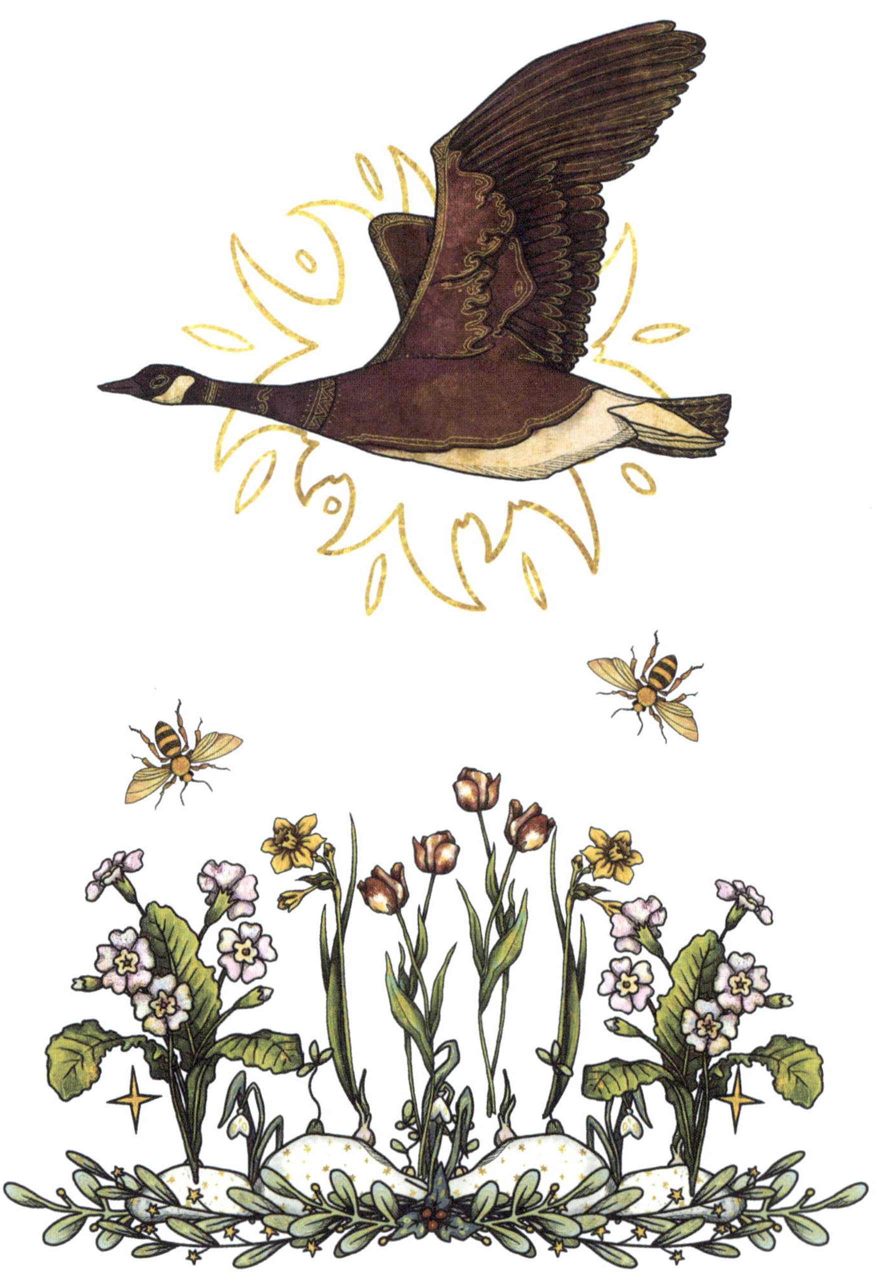

# *Spring*

The wild and greening land comes to life as winter recedes. Energy rises from the earth, drawn up by the strengthening sun, bringing a liveliness to the air. Spring is a time for celebrating, blessing what is reemerging, returning home, and blossoming for the first time—from the births of little ones to the embrace of new identities and the promise of bright possibilities. The land stirs awake and sings, transformed and renewed by what has been before, dreaming of possibilities in the brightening year.

In lands where cold lingers long past its welcome, you'll often find myths of the Old One of Winter who eventually returns back up to the mountain, into a cave, or beneath the waters, tired and ready to retreat or sometimes driven off by the raucous light of people singing in the spring—but always, *eventually*, leaving. Spring arrives, precious and quick, stirring up the sluggish currents of the land with vibrant flowers and returning birds, creating an ever-brightening cacophony of color and noise. Arms full of the quickening remedies of spring, we wake our bodies from winter's rest with everything from lymphatic tonics to warming digestives and emollient skin treatments.

Within traditional western herbalism, healing stories tell us spring is when the energies of water meet the energies of air, creating life-supporting dampness and warmth. Spring is also a time of archetypal childhood, the compass direction east, and the clarifying energy of the new moon. Guided by the increasing vitality of air, we stretch into spring through the breath, practicing our own spring movement and breathwork, while helping our homes breathe by opening windows and cleaning our spaces physically and energetically.

The increasing light stirs up energy in our bodies, and with increased energy comes nourishment needs differing from our winter practices, leading us to clear out what is no longer necessary in our lives and spaces, welcoming in what will better serve us instead. Spring and summer are also some of the busiest times for remedy-making, as we revel in the abundance the land offers, practicing our own engaged stewardship and kinship with the land in turn. The land stirs with energy, and we can find ourselves caught up in the excitement of the season or overwhelmed by the sudden influx of energy. So we turn to the land and our plant allies to help us center, rebuild our energetic stores, and become curious about what the season of healing might bring.

What forms will the dreams of winter take as wakefulness spreads across the spring land?

**Slow Winter, Soft Spring Breathwork**

*Find a comfortable position to relax into. I enjoy bringing my breathwork practice outside in spring so I can sit directly on the earth and have an easy view of the sky. Take a few soft, centering breaths. On your next outbreath try and extend your exhalation as long and slow as possible. Pause. On your inbreath, feel yourself pulling in soft, slow-spiraling energy from the earth below you. Continue in this pattern of breath for a count of nine (a single inbreath and outbreath is one count) or longer. As your breathwork comes to a close, let the soft energy settle all around you, like a comforting layer of light.*

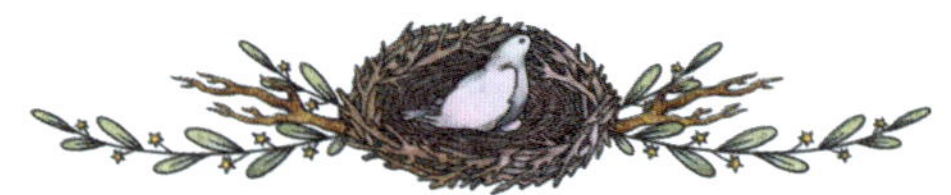

## The Gifts of Spring

### *Tenderness*

The start of spring is a liminal time. Momentum and growth expand swiftly after the long wait of winter, but are accompanied by such precarity of new life that we can feel vulnerable in all sorts of ways. I like to use the word *tenderness* to describe this particular and precious gift of spring. It embodies vulnerability and ease, uncertainty and softness, gentleness and courage. We all deserve to be welcomed into the world with tenderness, and while some of us experience being held gently in our early years, others have to seek out later the tenderness we weren't always afforded in our childhoods. Just like the early stages of growth in the garden, this is a time when the cycle of life can be too easily disrupted as young seedlings try to root securely in the soil, seeking out the nutrients to grow into robust plants later. That disruption of early growth not only shapes the land in interesting ways, but our own inner landscape, too.

Tenderness and its accompanying vulnerability and openness can make many of us squirm. Winter's harshness emphasizes our vulnerabilities and how interconnected we are with the world, how reliant we are on shelter built in warmer times, as well as food harvested and successfully stored to survive through lean months. For many of us, though, scarcity is not tied so much to the seasons as it is to paychecks, the whims of landlords, and a lack of free or affordable quality health care. Under the artifices of capitalism trying to convince us every day we are not cyclical creatures with cyclical needs, many of us experience a year full of winters, the landscapes of our bodies exhausted by endless scarcity, struggling to connect to winter's healing rest and the hope of spring. How do we let ourselves breathe into the opening of spring under these circumstances? Through the land, we seek out our tenderness, inviting spring into our lives with the knowing of our softest places, and recognizing winter's transformation into spring as the land reveals its longest-night dreams through flowers, tender grasses, tree buds, and birdsong. Through tenderness a path of strength and healing can be found between and through the seasons.

At first glance, tenderness might not be something we would associate with strength, healing, and robust health. Yet tenderness and being tender are essential to both healing and magickal work. Folks in my classes or consultations are often seeking to feel strong and empowered—which are wonderful things to strive for—and want to work with plants and practices to achieve just that. When I start suggesting practices about ease and gentleness, rest and tenderness, as well as openhearted vulnerability, reactions can range from disbelief to dismissiveness, often hiding an underlying and reasonable fear. To get tender with oneself is a process of being honest about what you need on a deep level. And after a lifetime of being *told* what we need, traumatic experiences, and/or cultural expectation of "appropriate" wants, tenderness can be an absolutely terrifying prospect. Seeking out and making space for the most tender parts of ourselves can often, at least initially, release a wellspring of grief as we acknowledge the ways our tenderness was neglected, taken advantage of, and hidden away. Yet meeting this grief with plant allies at our side and tenderness as our companion makes space for us to be gently and fiercely loved.

Spring comes in full of tenderness but somehow always makes it through to summer. We, too, can be tender and thriving like spring, our healing and magickal practices made that much richer because we know what our heart wants. What tenderness do you see when you look around the land? The tiniest of sprouts, the little buds on still bare branches, the way that sound returns to the land gleefully, unhesitantly, like a toddler exploring a new noise they've discovered they can make. Spring storms can test all of these tender edges, blowing away the protective leaf cover over seedlings, flooding meadows, downing trees. The weather jumps between unseasonably warm to sudden frosts, and we manage the multilayered weather with a variety of clothing and attitudes. Still, spring arrives, having been called in by winter's desire to retire, our bodies carrying the starry hope of long nights with us into the growing warmth of lengthening days.

One of the easiest places to find tenderness in our lives is through the dreams we keep close to our heart, hidden from the gaze of anyone but our most trusted companions. As winter wakes, dreams scatter like seeds on blustery spring winds. Our dreaming bodies begin to transform, too, as we imagine what a dream given a chance in the waking world might become. Some of us hide our dreams behind brambles, deep within mountain caverns, in unwelcoming arid landscapes—we are still learning to trust the soil. Others struggle to know where it is our dreams will best thrive. Our work in spring becomes learning to trust our own tender earth, to loosen up the tension of keeping our dreams safe from fears of failure, but ultimately unrealized, into something easeful and abundant. Plant allies like Dandelion (*Taraxacum officinale*) Lemon Balm (*Melissa officinalis*), Mugwort (*Artemisia vulgaris*) and Sage (*Salvia officinalis*) can help us explore new landscapes within and around us that are more hospitable to our dreams coming to life.

Cultivating a relationship with our own tender needs and those of our loved ones and community is a practice of curiosity and compassion, helping us to be


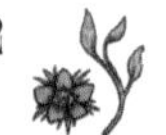

gentler and more welcoming of differences in those needs. We better understand what shelter we can build in our lives during the long bright months of summer when we have a clearer understanding of our vulnerability and tender desires; we are more able to set the boundaries needed in autumn to protect our tenderness; and in winter, tenderness becomes the light by which we find one another during the longest nights of the year. During spring, we can renew our commitment to the most vulnerable in our communities, finding folks still lost in the scarcity of winter, reseeding resources, and experimenting with ways we can be of service that are sustainable and life-affirming. Spring is a time to assess our winter pantries, finding what we have used up and what we still have in abundance to offer others from physical resources (e.g., herbal remedies, books, clothing), shareable skills (e.g., supporting young herbalists in setting up businesses, building garden boxes), and all variety of energetic, emotional, and technical services.

We can practice tender reciprocity with our friends, family, and beloved community, helping them make the transition from winter to spring and beyond, exploring how we create space for tenderness in our relationships and communities. What are the ways you create space—whether in your home, your classroom, your consultations, your community meetings, festivals, sacred gathering places, and beyond—for folks to soften their edges and open up to their tenderness?

When I am preparing for teaching, I focus on creating spaces that feel inviting, inclusive, and inspiring. I want folks to know what to expect from our time together through actions like sharing the event's schedule and where they can find amenities like restrooms, quiet spaces outside of the classroom for breaks, and places to find water, food, and tea. I always try to use accessible spaces and gentle lighting, request folks refrain from wearing heavy scents, make sure a variety of sitting options are available, and create the boundary of no videos or photography during the event so that no one has to worry about their private class experience becoming a public display. Of course, this is just a short list of choices I've made while asking myself, *How can I help my students show up to the tender needs of their curiosity and connection with our classroom community?*

Physically, at the end of winter and beginning of spring, we might be recovering from common illnesses brought on by the cold, dry air of winter in addition to prolonged exposure indoors with other people. It is an act of tenderness to acknowledge we need extra support, are still sick, or still recovering. The remedies made in spring work to protect us against illness later in the year so that when we do get sick we'll have a supply of lymphatic tonics, nourishing nervines, antihistamines, and digestives to feel better quicker.

## *Momentum*

Tenderness is the precursor to spring's second gift of momentum, drawing us out of the comfort of winter's stillness into the heartwinds of spring's return. Seedlings burst from the earth; buds ripen and bloom; birds fill the air with joyful noises after returning from their winter refuge; and the earth stretches out, bringing warmth to the land. From the embers of possibility kept burning through the long winter, we light candles and bonfires, drawing our dreams from the ethereal to the tangible. Not every dream will make it—surviving to spring is no guarantee that a dream will see summer. But the momentum of spring asks us, *Why not try?*

Through our tenderness we learn to recognize what we are most curious about, inspired by, and drawn to, pulling us into trying out, experimenting with, and seeking out the experiences we're excited by or feel increasingly necessary. Momentum is not a starting point but the result of energy being freed up and let loose to move in the way it feels most empowered to. The seedlings springing up throughout the land are not suddenly *there* but are able to grow because of the various processes of decay needed to create soil; the movement of water between land, sea, and sky; and seeds being freed from fruits and skins and pods by all sorts of interactions with animals, insects, fungi, and more. So too does our own momentum for growth, action, and rest arise from an interwoven landscape of experiences and our varying levels of self-awareness of that experience.

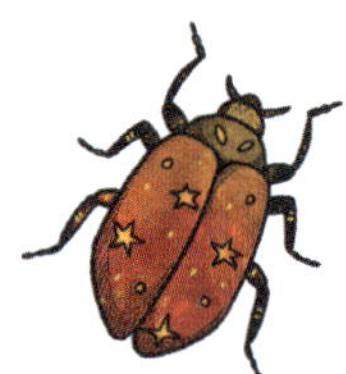

I try to help folks tap into their momentum from places of hope, delight, the joy of unburdening, and learning what it is their land-body wants and needs. I find community momentum gathers best where resources are being shared and exchanged, from libraries and learning collectives, seed and time banks, farmers markets, street fairs, block parties, and all sorts of free or low-cost public gatherings. Not only do I show up when I can in these spaces as a participant, volunteer, or collaborative organizer, but I make sure I can easily point my clients and community toward these spaces, helping them connect their inner landscapes with the people around them, letting one map flow into another.

Many of our spring plant allies work to wake us up, nourish us, and move energy by supporting the lymphatic system, our digestive health, and clearing out brain fog. The wild weedy plants growing in abundance in spring such as Dandelion (*Taraxacum officinale*), Cleavers (*Galium aparine*), and Calendula (*Calendula officinalis*) all move stagnant energy and create internal momentum within various body systems, making room for our dreams and getting swept up in (instead of swept under) the excitement of what might be possible for us and our communities. When sitting with folks looking for herbal support, I try to listen to not only where there might be a lack or hindrance of momentum, but where momentum is already present, however small a spark that might be, and how we can nourish its source. Very often, their momentum has led them to connect with plant allies, and simply introducing them to a few plants they resonate with can nurture that initial spark into a bright flame.

What we must be careful with in spring is recognizing that momentum and its older cousin manifestation are easily misused by voracious capitalist-driven consumerism hiding behind a thin veneer of spiritual empowerment. Momentum is not productivity or achievement, endless goal-setting and personal growth, but simply *movement*. It is the movement of the heart beating in our chest, the expansion and contraction of our lungs, our breath pulled in and pushed out, our blood flowing, and the electric transmissions of our synapses and nerves. Momentum is spring winds whipping across the land, snow melting and filling up rivers, clouds stirring up rain, bees rummaging among newly awakened flowers, the air filling up with scent and sound. Momentum is a song that calls us back to the land and out of our muddled stagnation, sparks our bravery, and helps us get carried by our dreams, not just held back by what we're afraid of.

With all this activity and energy so visible in the land and tugging at the edges of our own land-bodies, it can be all too easy to feel impatient at any perceived lack of momentum in our own life. We are presented with endless demands for our attention, labor, and whatever the latest iteration of productivity culture is. It can be easy to feel like we've fallen behind some arbitrary measure of success, distracting us from the real urgent needs of abundance like food, housing, health care, education, and art. We can be anxious that we're not "improving" fast enough through endless goals, thinking that once we achieve or purchase or are recognized for something *over there,* we'll finally be satisfied with who we are *right here*. The beauty of spring's momentum—an energy that we can carry with us throughout the year—is that it can help move us in the direction of our life-affirming, mental health–supporting, emotionally resilient goals. We just have to be wary of getting caught up in demands placed upon us instead of ones we have drawn up from our own deep wells of desire.

Sometimes momentum—and the possibilities of change and the unknown riding along with it—can summon fear from deep within us. Even though I love the magick springs bring, I can get caught up in the fear of what spring represents for me and wish for winter to last a little longer. Where I live spring is a short bridge to summer and months of heat that can lead to deadly fires, starkly underlying the existential terror of the climate emergency. Spring can generate in me a strong instinct to pack up my loved ones and move somewhere safer—an instinct passed down to me through generations of people who did pack up, who left, who tried to stay one step ahead of whatever was trying to tear them apart. It took me a while to recognize that while there is no safer space out there, I can cultivate a safer landscape within me while working collectively for a better future. So I let those voices of my ancestors run through me like spring waters coming down from the mountains, and I let myself get carried away, allowing them to shape me like water against my bone-rock-stone. Instead of drowning in anxiousness, I let myself float in currents of healing carrying their wisdom. What ancestral stories do you know you carry that shape your instincts around safety and security?


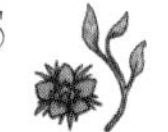

Carried by these inner instincts, I listen to the waters of my body, their currents shaped by my own lived experiences and passed on to me through generations trying to stay alive. Without these waters, I could not live, and on these waters, I have been carried, imagining every one of us as a river come ashore until we return again to the sea. So I play in the waters; I let the river of time run through me; I don't try to hold on to it. I let the waters flow, removing as many impediments as possible, allowing my inner landscape to be nourished, giving the fauna and flora of the river edges room to flourish with life.

One of the most powerful ways to connect with the watery energy of the body is by working with the vagus nerve. The long inner river known as the vagus nerve travels down from the ocean consciousness of our brain through the vast lands of our heart and into the delta of our digestive system. As spring stirs up energy in our own bodies, the vagus nerve becomes energized with the growth of light and heat. It's an incredible pathway of connective energy, modulating function between body systems and supporting the flow of the parasympathetic nervous system to rest, digest, and repair. Some people have vagus nerve waterways close to the surface, and disruptions to our river are felt quickly even if we aren't always aware of the cause. For others, our waterways run deep underground, and while it seems we are less easy to disrupt, it can be, in turn, harder to identify what we are experiencing and feeling—nothing disturbs us, but also nothing seems to aid or move us either. To support the nervous system and the work of the vagus nerve, we can turn to spring plant allies like Milky Oat (*Avena sativa*), Lemon Balm (*Melissa officinalis*), and Ashwagandha (*Withania somnifera*) as well as grounding and centering practices.

The momentum of spring is carried by the elemental energy of air, returning like migrating birds to the waking land. Air is energizing, electric, and life-supporting, moving through us as breath, creating sound, and traveling across the land as wind that can topple trees as easily as it can bring cool relief on a hot day. Within Western esoteric tradition, air is the element of the mind, referring to both the energetic mind of consciousness and intelligence as well as the physical brain. To work with air and the complexity of the conscious and subconscious mind is to explore what makes life meaningful, the intangible boundaries we construct and deconstruct as a species between ourselves and all of existence, and what it is we need to feel fully ourselves. In traditional western herbalism, the seat of air is in the liver and in modern western herbalism the seat of air is in the nervous system as well and shows up as Tension in the body and the land. Herbs like Skullcap (*Scutellaria lateriflora*), Sage (*Salvia officinalis*), Peppermint (*Mentha piperita*), Lavender (*Lavandula* spp.), and Lemon Balm (*Melissa officinalis*) all possess strong air energy and can help us connect to the air of our land-body.

As the energy of water flows into the energy of air, supporting the nervous system is one way we can work with the strong elemental air energy spring brings. An increase in air brings inspiration and clarity—both essential to our tenderness and momentum—but when we have difficulty processing air energy, we can feel frazzled, irritated, tense, scattered, disconnected, and/or impatient. Our symptoms sometimes seem random as the winds shift and change, so I recommend turning to grounding and centering practices to find your equilibrium:

- Getting the bare skin of your land-body on the earth to ground energy
- Visualizing yourself as a tree with roots going down into the earth
- Bodywork and herbal oil massage
- Engaging movement that requires your full attention
- Going on a date with partners, friends, loved ones focused on enjoying being in each other's company
- Working with roots, such as Dandelion (*Taraxacum officinale*), and nutritive herbs, such as Nettles (*Urtica dioica*), and fresh spring herbs as daily tonics

## Spring Inquiry

*What is my spring story?*

*What does spring feel, look, smell, and taste like in my body?*

*What does spring feel, look, smell, and taste like in the land around me?*

*Where am I feeling tender in my life and my body?*

*What is the tenderness I see across the land and in my communities?*

*How would I grow if I didn't feel rushed?*

*Where am I feeling momentum in my life and my body?*

*What momentum do I see in the land around me?*

*When do I feel the most free to follow where my energy takes me?*

## Herbs for the Spring Body

Within traditional western herbalism, spring is a time of damp and moisture, moving from the cold water of winter into the increasingly warm air of spring. We see this in the land through frozen ice and snow melting, giving way to water flowing and filling up the land, combined with the heat of the warming sun, bringing about a state of damp fecundity. The return of moisture alleviates the dry brittleness of winter, and the increasing warmth draws the energy of the land up and outward. Within our apothecaries we can support the energy of spring through lymphatic and digestive tonics, respiratory plants to help us breathe easy, vitamin- and mineral-rich daily tonics, as well as astringents and emollients to manage the flow and movement of moisture throughout our bodies.

As the energy of water recedes and the energy of air emerges across the land, spring helps us understand the sources of beneficial and less desirable Tension in our life. While we need Tension to move our muscles and maintain structures, set boundaries, and focus, an excess of Tension can lead to too much stress, an inability to relax deeply, and all the accompanying symptoms of headaches, indigestion, irritation, and anxiety. In the extreme, too much Tension can lead to burnout and adrenal fatigue. Though Tension can be a challenging tissue state to balance, it also effectively draws our focus to the area of our inner landscape in deepest need of healing—where we are trying to keep it all together so we can hide away our most tender places. As excellent allies of stress relief, many herbs alleviate Tension. We can turn to relaxants and nervous system tonics like Milky Oat (*Avena sativa*), Rose (*Rosa* spp.), and Skullcap (*Scutellaria lateriflora*), combined with herbs addressing secondary symptoms like Fennel (*Foeniculum vulgare*) for indigestion or Wood Betony (*Betonica officinalis*) for headaches, to dissipate Tension and bring us into a relaxed state of being.

As a season associated with childhood and children, not only is spring a great time to work with herbs like Lemon Balm (*Melissa officinalis*), Chamomile (*Matricaria chamomilla*), and Catnip (*Nepeta cataria*) in making remedies for the little ones in your life, but it can be a wonderful time to do some gentle inner-child work for your own healing needs. You can also work with the growing tide of energy in the land by tending to your nervous system and focusing on your own personal riverway, the vagus nerve.

The land is full of dreams coming into being during spring, so it's important to connect with plants that support our dreaming body, our bravery, and our joyful expansiveness, especially if the winter has been long and hard. Mugwort (*Artemisia vulgaris*) is a beloved herbal elder within the traditional Western herbalist *materia medica*, honored as the "Oldest of Herbs" and a long-trusted guide within the land of dreams.[1] But any plant ally can be a dream ally, a bravery booster, an elixir of joy—spring just happens to be an energetically auspicious time to explore who these allies might be and grow into a relationship with them.


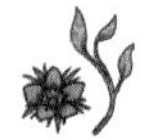

# Spring Plant Allies

## Lemon Balm

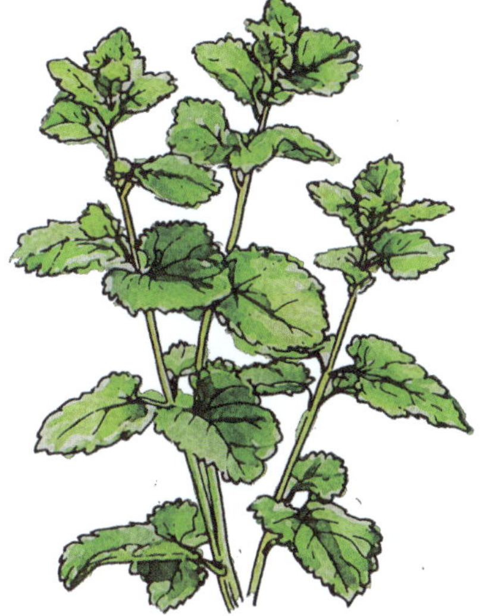

*(Melissa officinalis)*

**Common + Folk Names:** Balm, bee balm, dropsy plant, heart's delight, melissa

**Elements:** Water, air

**Zodiac Signs:** Embodies the energy of Cancer, Libra, and Pisces. A remedy for Aries, Cancer, Leo, Virgo, Sagittarius, and Aquarius.

**Planets:** Jupiter, Mercury, Venus

**Moon Phase:** Full moon

**Parts Used:** Aerial parts

**Habitat:** Native of southern Europe, but widely cultivated

**Growing Conditions:** Full sun to partial shade with moderate watering and well-drained soil

**Collection:** Collect leaves and flowers throughout spring and summer.

**Flavor:** Sour

**Temperature:** Cool

**Moisture:** Dry

**Tissue States:** Heat, Stagnation, Tension

**Actions:** Antibacterial, antidepressant, antihistamine, anti-inflammatory, antioxidant, antispasmodic, antiviral, aromatic, carminative, cholagogue, diaphoretic, digestive, emmenagogue, febrifuge, hepatic, nervine, sedative, digestive, vasodilator

**Contraindications:** May interfere with thyroid medications. Avoid in cases of glaucoma as Lemon Balm may increase eye pressure.

**Dosage:** Standard dosage

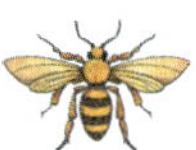

I love Lemon Balm for its ability to hold our tenderness while encouraging our momentum—but at a pace and rhythm that feels good and joyful to our inner landscape.

Within traditional western herbalism, Lemon Balm has long historical use as a spirit-elevating, body systems–energizing, nervous system–nourishing vitality tonic. English herbalist Thomas Bartram notes that Lemon Balm is used "[t]o strengthen the brain in its resistance to shock and stress," as well as its effectiveness in "protect[ing] the cerebrum" and treating "autonomic disorders—an action similar to modern tranquilisers . . . usually combined with Peppermint."[2] Acting on the limbic system of the brain (instinct and mood), it is gently sedating and useful for all kinds of hyperactivity, tension, and nervousness.

I like to think of Lemon Balm as an herb for overextension that leads to burnout. I often suggest Lemon Balm for sensitive folks and those who are in the healing fields, since I find it helps us open up as conduits of healing energy without resulting in exhaustion from always trying to assist others. The herb is similarly useful for folks of all ages struggling under systems that don't support their inherent high-energy expressiveness and/or neurodiversity. Lemon Balm can and should be taken over an extended period of time and can be easily added to most herbal blends.

In my experience, Lemon Balm has been one of the most reliable herbs for alleviating stress and restoring joy. Drinking Lemon Balm tea over a few months can support our ability to heal after traumatic events but also from years of accumulated stress. This herb is also good for all times of transition, from postpartum to school-life changes to relocating, new relationships, and shifts in identity. Lemon Balm also helps us manage social anxiety, for example,

when there is a need for connection but sometimes difficulty in showing up in community spaces.

Lemon Balm alleviates colds and flu as well as aids in recovery from debilitating illness. It's a great herb for children's fevers—consider combining with Elderflower and Elderberry (*Sambucus nigra*), Chamomile (*Matricaria chamomilla*), and Peppermint (*Mentha piperita*). Alternatively, use as a bath for those children resistant to taking tea. It is also helpful for children who are prone to anxiety about school, exams, and general performance and can be drunk as a tea before bed to alleviate nightmares.

As a carminative, Lemon Balm is excellent in cases of spasms along the digestive tract, relieving flatulence and indigestion, and cases of "nervous stomach" when an upset stomach is caused by tension, depression, and stress. Its sour taste awakens the energies of the liver and indicates vitamin C and other nutrients are present, helping to tonify body systems. Headaches, migraines, insomnia, and other anxiety-induced symptoms are soothed by Lemon Balm. In cases of hyperthyroidism, Lemon Balm has been shown to have hormone-regulating effects to rebalance thyroid function as well as being a gentle cardio tonic useful for regulating heart rhythms.

Apply Lemon Balm topically as an herbal oil or liniment for its antihistamine properties. You can also make an antiviral salve to apply to herpes simplex lesions. It's a great plant to add to herbal steams to clear up congestion and relax spasmodic coughs. Use in mouthwashes for ulcers, gum infections, and general toothache.

### Seasonal Uses

Lemon Balm is one of my favorite spring tonic herbs and can be added to daily teas to support general well-being and for its antihistamine qualities. In summer, Lemon Balm in teas can help us to stay grounded in the moment, strengthening our internal compass to guide us toward healing community connections while alleviating the stress this season can bring around social expectations. Add Lemon Balm to your cold and flu blends in autumn as preventative care, during illness, and in the recovery period. Adding Lemon Balm to winter teas and baths invites warmth and hope into the darkest part of the year.

## Magickal Uses

Lemon Balm's Latin genus *Melissa* connects the herb to the ancient bee priestesses of Greece. The *Melissae* or "bees" were priestesses of the goddess Demeter (or Venus), and Melissa was also another name for the moon goddess Artemis. Bees are messengers of the goddess, and the herb can be used in all spells of communication and intuition. Lemon Balm can be employed in rituals strengthening relationships of all kinds. One of my favorite herbs for introducing the magick of plants to children, Lemon Balm makes a beautiful moon or sun tea with calming properties.

## The Lemon Balm Personality

The Lemon Balm person tends to be nervous and on edge. Panic attacks can be an unfortunately familiar experience, often rearing up when any stressful change occurs in their life. Such constant worry and stress can lead to mental fatigue and burnout, making the effort to seek out support, healing modalities, and skill sets to bring much needed relief that much harder. Even though many Lemon Balm folk operate under an incredible weight of anxiety, they are often the helpers and givers in their relationships—they not only worry for themselves but about everyone else, too. This brings about a state of physical and emotional tension that can lead to debilitating burnout if not tended to. While one of the first goals for Lemon Balm folks is to accept they are deserving of care no matter what, the path to that sort of wisdom often needs support to open up to Lemon Balm. Lemon Balm folks need a release valve, and the plant helps to reconnect the heart to the head, delivering messages of calm when all seems topsy-turvy. One of the most healing actions that Lemon Balm folks can take is finding a way back into community, learning how to be seen and held by others, and instead of being isolated by the static of their anxiety, find their harmony with those who love them.


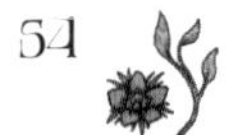

# Rose

*(Rosa spp.)*

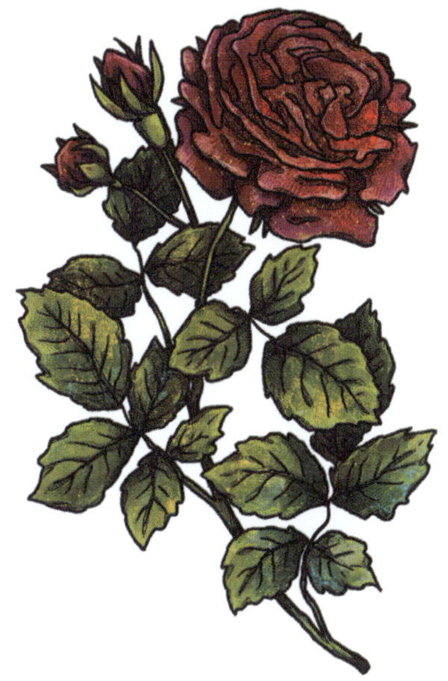

**Common + Folk Names:** Queen of flowers, rosa, satapatri, witch's briar, thorn mother, oginii-waabigwan

**Elements:** Water, air, fire

**Zodiac Signs:** Embodies the energy of Taurus and Libra. A remedy for all signs.

**Planets:** Venus, Jupiter, Mars, moon

**Moon Phase:** Full moon

**Parts Used:** Flowers, hips, roots

**Habitat:** There are 47 species of the *Rosa* genus growing wild in Europe and 10,000 varieties, both wild and cultivated, worldwide.

**Growing Conditions:** Partial shade to full sun with frequent watering

**Collection:** Collect rosehips before flowering. Collect flowers in the spring and summer.

**Flavor:** Bitter, sweet, astringent

**Temperature:** Cooling

**Moisture:** Moist (flower + seed), Dry (hip + root)

**Tissue States:** Heat, Relaxation, Cold

**Actions:** Diaphoretic, carminative, probiotic, hepatoprotective, emmenagogue, reproductive tonic, aphrodisiac, aperient, decongestant, febrifuge, nervine, anxiolytic, antidepressant, anti-inflammatory, astringent, hemostatic, antimicrobial, antidepressant, analgesic, vulnerary, deodorant. *Flower:* Anodyne, antibacterial, antidepressant, antifungal, anti-inflammatory, antiseptic, antispasmodic, antiviral, aphrodisiac, aromatic, astringent, blood tonic, cardiotonic, carminative, decongestant, diuretic, emmenagogue, expectorant, hemostatic, hepatic, kidney tonic, laxative, refrigerant, sedative. *Hip:* Antibacterial, anti-inflammatory, antimutagenic, antioxidant, antiviral, astringent, blood tonic, cardiotonic, digestive, diuretic (mild), emmenagogue, kidney tonic, laxative, nutritive, stimulant, tonic. *Seed:* Diuretic, laxative. *Root:* Astringent, carminative.

**Contraindications:** Caution during pregnancy and while nursing

**Dosage:** Standard dosage

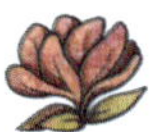

Rose is one of the elder plants of our home planet, used medicinally for thousands of years, and a beloved ancestor of our herbal practice. The herb helps us tap into ancestral wisdom, honor the ancient animal nature of our sensitivity, and learn how to unfold into our gifts just as a many-petaled Rose unfolds into maturity.

As a sweet medicine that calms the nervous system, Rose assists with memory and promotes clarity of mind, heart, and spirit by connecting all three centers of experience. Within Ayurveda, Rose is considered a *rasayana* (rejuvenative tonic) and *medhya* (brain tonic and nervine) for all of the doshas. The Anishinaabe have a myth about Rose that teaches that "[t]he sight and smell of a rose are here to remind us of the harmony inherent in our world. The thorns are there to keep us mindful of greed that endangers the balance and thereby endangers the whole of creation."[3]

Rose is an essential remedy for imbalances arising from excess inflammation. The flower relieves pain from heat and inflammation, including gastritis, peptic ulcers, and cooling an overheated liver. Rose's cooling qualities also alleviate the heat that can accompany autoimmune conditions and assist topically and internally with arthritic pain, improving flexibility of movement. Use as a remedy for fluid imbalances that lead to depletion of energy and blood in the body, including diarrhea, excess bleeding, and the accumulation of fluids.

Rose prevents and alleviates colds and can also be used in the case of flu, sore throats, excess mucus, and coughs, including bronchitis. Rose is an uplifting, soothing, and nourishing medicine for those with weakened vitality, including children, elders, and people in recovery from illness. For fluid imbalances Rose can be effective in cases of an overactive bladder, bed-wetting, night sweats, and general excess excretion of fluids. Excessive menstruation is eased by a strong tea of dried Rose, and the herb is also useful for uterine spasms and cramping. A vaginal douche can relieve infection, inflammation, and conditions such as vaginitis and thrush. As an astringent, Rose can be useful for diarrhea and internal hemorrhage as well as acting as a healing herb in postpartum sitz baths.

As a digestive aid, Rose has wonderful probiotic qualities and supports healthy gut flora. Use Rose during and after taking antibiotics to rebuild gut flora as it encourages the growth of beneficial bacteria while countering harmful pathogens. As a clearing herb, Rose improves circulation and promotes healthy blood flow, breaks up kidney stones and helps the kidneys process toxins, and relieves brain fog.

As an aphrodisiac, Rose is an opener—it opens the heart and body to healing experiences with oneself and others. Like many aphrodisiacs, Rose has nervine qualities that relax the body into a place of connected intimacy. For those seeking fertility support, Rose has also been shown to increase sperm count.

In addition to the powder and juice of Rose, a Rose honey can be a topical treatment for inflammation, rashes, wounds, ulcers, acne, herpes, and similar skin imbalances. My favorite form of Rose skincare is rosewater, which adds and maintains water in the skin and can be used as a mild antiseptic for first-aid needs. Use as a mouthwash for ulcers and bleeding gums. Rose vinegar or a strong tea is especially cooling and repairing for the skin after prolonged sun exposure. Apply externally on the eyes as a soothing compress to relieve eyestrain and conjunctivitis and improve vision.

### Seasonal Uses

In spring Rose skincare recipes rejuvenate winter skin. A Rose herbal oil can loosen up stiff joints, waking the body up to the new season. In summer, use rosewater, a strong Rose tea, or Rose vinegar for after-sun care, and keep Rose honey or Rose petal powder handy for stings, bumps, and bruises. In autumn rosehips are a great addition to tea to prevent colds and flu. Add Rose petals to teas and desserts during winter to gladden the heart and as a digestive aid so that the body can rest deeply during the darkest part of the year.

## Magickal Uses

The Rose is a symbol of many ancient goddesses, including Ishtar, Isis, and Aphrodite. The flower also has a special relationship to Sappho and lesbians as it is from Sappho that Rose received the name "Queen of Flowers."[4] Use Rose in spells and charms for love, desire, charm, and attraction. Add the petals to your dream pillow to dream of love. Rose is a great plant ally for those desiring to deepen their spiritual study and experience. Add to charms of mirth, reverence, and joy. Use in charms of secrecy ("under the rose . . ."). Use in handfasting rituals for divine blessing of the union. Thorns can be included in charms of protection. Rose tea awakens psychic visions and connects us to our intuitive heart-knowings.

## The Rose Personality

The Rose personality has lost their spark of desire. They might have trouble sleeping, be restless and exhausted, and ultimately not have enough energy to explore their worlds either physically or philosophically. The desire to create and experience life and relationships of all kinds is low; their vitality stagnant. What they *think* they should be doing dominates their thoughts more than what they *want* to be doing. Sometimes they are not even sure they know what they want to be doing. Many Rose folks experience a disconnection in relationships, creating distance between themselves and those they love. For those who've been in this state of exhaustion for a while, their brain and heart fog can be punctured by sudden overwhelming feelings of despair, like they are living without a light in the dark. Sometimes, unresolved anger simmers deep below the surface—Rose teaches us how to use both our thorns and petals to set up boundaries and supportive spaces to express how we really feel. Working with Rose helps folk reconnect to their wildness, their fierceness, and their determination to know and name their heart's desires. Rose helps folks to dream and want and feel and move closer to the relationships that feel whole and holy, closing the distance between themselves and the people, places, and creatures they love. Ultimately, Rose connects folks back to the secret excitement of mystery, where it is safe to express desire and seek it out. The profound gift of Rose folks is the ability to name desire, honor it in others, and shine like a fiery, welcoming, and protective light wherever they go.


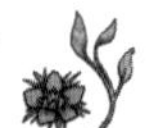

# Skullcap

*(Scutellaria lateriflora)*

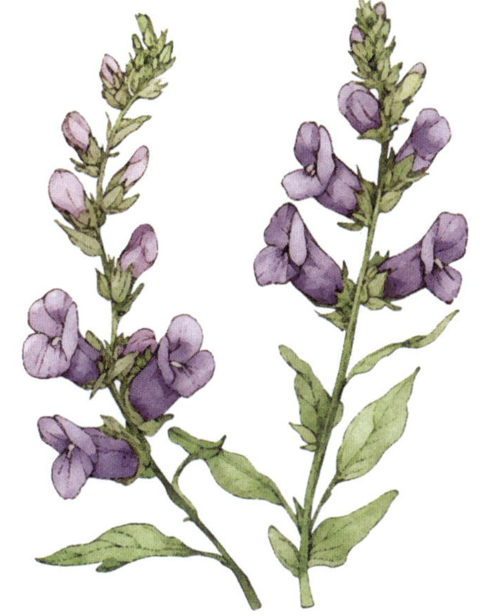

**Common + Folk Names:** Mad dog weed, madweed, Quaker's hat or bonnet, blue pimpernel, helmet flower

**Elements:** Water, air

**Zodiac Signs:** Embodies and remedies the energy of Gemini and Virgo

**Planets:** Moon, Saturn, Mercury, Neptune, Pluto

**Moon Phase:** Dark moon, full moon

**Parts Used:** Leaf and flower

**Habitat:** Native to North America and Eurasia

**Growing Conditions:** Full sun with plenty of space and not overly rich soil

**Collection:** Summer, before flowering

**Flavor:** Bitter

**Temperature:** Cold

**Moisture:** Dry

**Tissue States:** Tension, Heat

**Actions:** Anodyne, antibacterial, antispasmodic, astringent, anxiolytic, bitter, brain tonic, cardiotonic, diuretic, febrifuge, vasodilator, hypotensive, nervine, sedative, spinal cord tonic

**Contraindications:** There are mixed opinions on Skullcap and pregnancy. While it has been safely used by generations of pregnant folk, as with any herbs during pregnancy and postpartum, you should always consult your herbalist before use. Caution is needed for large doses in conjunction with CNS depressants such as alcohol, antidepressants, and antiepileptics.

**Dosage:** Small doses are quite effective and recommended with Skullcap: 3–10 drops up to three times daily of a 1:5 alcohol extract or 1 teaspoon of herb per cup of water.

☽●☾

One way we connect to the land within and around us is listening to and aligning with the stories of our own inner seasons. Skullcap is an ally for those of us learning how to listen in ways we haven't before, helping us to reconnect to stories of healing.

A powerful nervine, Skullcap restores strength to an overwhelmed nervous system, from relieving spasms and nerve pain to cultivating calm. It is one of my favorite plant allies for folks with busy brains and a lot of distracting inner chatter. For nervousness, fear, and a sense of being overwhelmed, Skullcap stimulates the brain to produce more endorphins. The herb is a beautiful brain tonic, helping us develop mental clarity and bringing a deep sense of wellness and peace to the nervous system. Too many of us live under systems and cultures glorifying overwork and excess productivity, ostracizing and punishing those who fall outside of the very narrow definition of what is valuable. Skullcap, with its message of balance and developing awareness between what we're thinking and what we're feeling, helps us disconnect from staying constantly busy and stimulated by tuning in to our internal land-based rhythms.

Skullcap assists with healthy sleep patterns and is an excellent ally for those suffering from insomnia, especially when there is difficulty shutting off the busy chatter of a restless mind. The wisdom of Skullcap returns us not only to a state of mental peace but dignity as we reassess what pressures are appropriate and inappropriate in our life. Skullcap makes a wonderful tea, blended with other plants like Rose (*Rosa* spp.) and Lemon Balm (*Melissa officinalis*), to end community meetings and gatherings with, supporting folks to depart feeling a gentle communion with one another.

Skullcap can be used for a variety of nervous conditions and imbalances stemming from hyperactivity, including ADHD, anxiety, hypertension, nervous


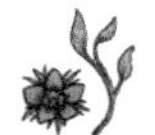

exhaustion, neuralgia, and premenstrual tension. Irritability is a big indicator for Skullcap as the plant helps release the buildup of frustration. The herb is a great ally for withdrawal from everything from caffeine, tranquilizers, and antidepressants to social media, gaming, and emerging forms of online addiction. Skullcap is useful in recovery periods from things that have generated prolonged stress, including illness and addiction.

Herbalist Karen M. Rose describes the energy of Skullcap as a "stern caregiver and parent . . . a fierce protective force that grounds an overactive nervous system," which is one of the reasons folks who carry so much fear and tension feel held by Skullcap.[5] Indications for Skullcap include the collapse of the ability to hide nervous tension—folks don't feel able to protect their tenderness from the world, resulting in increased fear and anxiety. Daily small doses over many months can be a helpful reset, assisting us in feeling embodied in our thoughts, dreams, and possibilities.

There are not many traditional topical uses for Skullcap, but I do add it to anxiety- and stress-alleviating bath blends and find it useful for skin recovery from all sorts of weather conditions (sun exposure, high winds, and dryness of both summer and winter).

### Seasonal Uses

In spring, Skullcap in herb and flower essence form supports the nervous system from the slowness of winter to the busyness of spring. For summer, make a sun recovery blend by brewing a quart of Skullcap tea, letting it cool to room temperature, and using as a body rinse or compress. Add Skullcap to topical treatments in autumn to recover from a long season of sun, protect the skin from the increasing cold and dryness, and nourish the nervous system from the outside in. During the winter Skullcap can be added to cold and flu blends as well as used before and during social gatherings to stay grounded and centered.

### Magickal Uses

Just as the herb is used to calm nervous conditions in the body, Skullcap can be used in rituals and spells for promoting peace and calm. Use post-meditation or after waking up from an intense dream or nightmare to ground and center. During trancework, journeying, and astral projection, Skullcap helps keep the spirit secured to the body so that it is able to find its way back. Skullcap is also an herb of oaths and binding contracts from business agreements to romantic unions. Skullcap has an affinity for the equinoxes, supporting us in transitioning from the bright half of the year to the dark half and back again.

### The Skullcap Personality

The Skullcap personality is easy to spot—their energy is intense, their muscles tight, and their minds busy. Often, their brow is furrowed, even when they are young children, as they are intensely occupied by their inner worlds. Energetic and quick, they can appear restless or overactive, which they sometimes are, but many Skullcap folk are purposefully busy and often happily engaged with whatever project or imaginative game they are pursuing. These are kids who enjoy problem-solving in their play—whether puzzles or saving the galaxy from certain doom—but often tend toward more nervous energy and fears in private moments even if they appear brave and confident in their play and relationships.

Skullcap folks can have a hard time feeling present in their bodies and can experience moments of disorientation—whether dizzy spells or struggling to find their physical edges. They have to be very careful about frequent burnout and making sure they take regular time off from their intense periods of thinking and doing. The great gift of Skullcap folk is that they have an incredible capacity to remain focused on the theoretical, impossible, and seemingly unattainable, bringing all into the range of the accessible for themselves and their community. Skullcap helps them to experience the balance necessary to play their part in saving the galaxy *and* get enough rest.



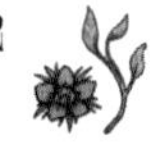

# The Spring Apothecary

## Waking Up from Winter: Brain Fog & Brain Tonics

### *Herbal Actions*

*Nootropics, nervines, and adaptogens along with herbs for digestive health to support the brain-gut axis*

Winter hopefully brought some much-needed slowness and rest to your life, and just like getting up in the morning after a long night's sleep, waking up from the winter months can take time. I like to reach for herbs that support brain health and mental clarity, helping to sweep away the cobwebs of winter to best enjoy the energy of spring.

**Ashwagandha (*Withania somnifera*):** An ally for folks dealing with brain fog and general stressed-based cognitive issues, Ashwagandha calms the nervous system, brings us back into our bodies, and starts the process of restorative nervous system healing. Indications include patterns of overwork, chronic illness, chronic anxiety, painful joints, muscle spasms, and general excess tension (i.e., trying to hold it all together when you are long overdue for an extended period of rest).

**Ginkgo (*Ginkgo biloba*):** Ginkgo is an especially wonderful ally to elders, but it can be used by all ages to support longevity, including improving memory and cognitive function, and protecting against cognitive impairment. Indications include poor memory, dizziness, and depression.

**Gotu Kola (*Centella asiatica*):** Gotu Kola improves memory and elevates the mood by moving energy between the hemispheres of the brain. Indications can be folks with post-traumatic stress disorder (PTSD), including marginalized folks experiencing the battle fatigue of simply existing on a daily basis, highly sensitive folks, as well as general care for the senior brain.

**Lemon Balm (*Melissa officinalis*):** My favorite ally for alleviating brain fog and promoting mental clarity, Lemon Balm brings joy and supports our ability to feel integrated with the world instead of overrun by it—something that can be especially useful between the slowness of winter and acceleration of spring. Indications include brain fog connected to social burnout or the precipice of social burnout (including social media–driven fear of missing out), nervous anxiety, and worry that results in insomnia and/or digestive issues (e.g., a nervous stomach).

**Milky Oat (*Avena sativa*):** A great nervous system tonic for those feeling exhausted and not ready to be doing much of anything, much less transitioning into a new season. Indications include recovering from an extended period of illness (including seasonal affective disorder), information overload, compassion fatigue, and premenstrual and menstrual brain fog.

**Sage (*Salvia officinalis*):** A classic brain tonic, Sage is known as an herb of wisdom, promoting mental clarity and discernment. Indications include headache when the head feels heavy and congested, brain fog that causes issues with short-term memory, and a general lack of energy and healthy tone and tension.

## The Internal Fire: Nourishing Digestion

### *Herbal Actions*

*Bitters, cholagogues, antispasmodic, anti-inflammatory, carminative, and nervine*

One of the most important ways of supporting health from a traditional western herbalism perspective is by supporting the digestive fire or metabolic processes of the body. After the long stretch of cold, in the spring we want to rekindle digestive effectiveness as we become more active on longer and warmer days. Finding the right digestive herbs for your constitution can take a bit of effort (which is why working with an herbalist one-on-one can be so valuable—you deserve such support), but when you find your digestive plant allies, it can be life-changing.

**Calendula (*Calendula officinalis*):** Deeply reparative to the digestive system, Calendula restores the digestive tract as well as clears out congestion in the gut. Indications for Calendula include signs of damp heat such as swollen glands,



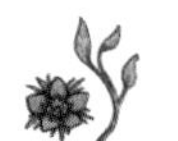

congestion in both the digestive tract and upper respiratory system, a feeling of overfullness, bloating, fatigue, and gas after meals, as well as thirst but dehydration.

**Chamomile (*Matricaria chamomilla*):** This is one of my favorite late spring, early summer digestive tonics that I especially like recommending to highly sensitive people who tend to get upset stomachs when experiencing disruption to their routine—including struggling with seasonal change. Chamomile is also great for folks with an overactive or fast digestion. Indications include digestive cramping, diarrhea, gas, and general crankiness.

**Dandelion (*Taraxacum officinale*):** The roots are a good overall spring tonic, waking up our winter bodies to the new season, while the leaves are particularly helpful for edema, warming up and moving out cold, stagnant water. Indications include water retention, constipation, slow digestion, gas, and indigestion headaches.

**Fennel (*Foeniculum vulgare*):** A good choice for slow and spasmodic digestion brought on by excess tension. Fennel rebuilds digestive fire, pulling energy down and out of the body (helping to alleviate the high and tight energy caused by tension). Indications include nausea and vomiting, food poisoning, and general lack of digestive fluids, which can cause constipation, dry stools, and hemorrhoids.

**Ginger (*Zingiber officinale*):** Ginger is a good choice for cold and damp digestion. The herb strengthens digestive fire, promotes the production of digestive fluids, and alleviates cramping. Indications include lack of appetite, nausea, high and tight energy, swelling, and spasms in the gut.

**Peppermint (*Mentha piperita*):** A great herb for digestive issues arising from stress and nervous conditions. Indications include cramping, headaches from digestive tension, lack of appetite, and distension.

**Rose (*Rosa* spp.):** A helpful ally when it comes to supporting the gut microbiome, Rose acts as a prebiotic as well as supporting digestion through promoting the production of bile. Indications include poor digestion, overactive and hot digestion leading to diarrhea, and gastritis.

**Rosemary (*Salvia rosmarinus*):** Rosemary assists with digestive complaints by supporting liver and gallbladder functions. The herb is antioxidant-rich, strengthening to the metabolism, warming to the stomach, and helping with the assimilation of nutrients. Indications include cold digestion resulting in gurgling, wet gas, and heaviness after meals.

**Sage (*Salvia officinalis*):** A gentle bitter, Sage helps us process and digest fats and nutrients. It can be particularly supportive in clearing out pathogens from the gut, including *E. coli*. Indications include cramping and signs of cold digestion (see Rosemary).

## The Body in Motion: Supporting the Lymph Nodes

### *Herbal Actions*

*Lymphatic, alterative, anti-inflammatory, and astringent*

Some of the first herbs to spring up after winter are those supporting lymphatic health, helping to drain congested lymphs and reduce overall inflammation, allowing our bodies to settle into a comfortable equilibrium. Often considered weeds by the general public, these herbs can be a beautiful and inexpensive way to access herbal medicine.

**Calendula (*Calendula officinalis*):** If you're in a state of lymphatic congestion, Calendula can be a beautiful ally. The bright flowers chase out shadows of sluggishness and promote lymphatic drainage and circulation. Indications include damp heat, rashes, and slow-healing wounds.

**Chickweed (*Stellaria media*):** A good lymph tonic in general, Chickweed is particularly indicated when signs of excess damp are present , such as wet coughs and runny noses. Chickweed has a short shelf life when dried, so fresh is best.

**Cleavers (*Galium aparine*):** These sweet and sticky herbs support the activity of white blood cells clearing out congestion in our lymph nodes. These are best taken fresh either as a tea or blended into smoothies.

**Dandelion (*Taraxacum officinale*):** Dandelion repairs and supports the filtering systems of our body, including our liver, kidneys, digestive tract, and lymph nodes. The herb promotes the production of lymphocytes, which makes it a wonderful lymph tonic throughout late winter and early spring. Indications include swollen lymphs, water retention, and sluggish digestion.

**Echinacea (*Echinacea purpurea*):** For more serious cases of inflammation and infection, Echinacea can be a useful, short-term ally. While Echinacea is great for stimulating the immune system for acute conditions, it should be avoided for chronic conditions and only taken up to one week at a time. Indications include tonsillitis, fever, and mastitis.

**Ocotillo (*Fouquieria splendens*):** Ocotillo is another good general lymph tonic especially when there are indications of indigestion and general digestive stagnation that have led to conditions such as hemorrhoids, eczema, and other signs of poor circulation.

## Balance: Managing Seasonal Allergies

### *Herbal Actions*

*Anti-inflammatory, antihistamine, anticatarrhal, and respiratory tonics*

There are so many herbs that are generally useful for allergies and helping the body be less reactive and inflammatory during allergen-abundant times like spring. My caveat about herbs and allergies is that this is an area of practice where most folks benefit from working one-on-one with a local herbalist specializing in allergy care to identify your particular reactivity because (a) allergies can be tricky to figure out and the individualized care of a practitioner can be essential to solving the puzzle, (b) there are often layers of reactivity (including food allergies and neuroplastic reactivity) that need exploring, and (c) a local herbalist can help you work with local herbs, which is often very beneficial with allergies. The following are a great place to start and generally protective against seasonal allergies, helping the body move from winter to spring.

**Dandelion (*Taraxacum officinale*):** Dandelion remedies made during the spring carry the energy of the season throughout the year. A wonderful general ally for allergies, Dandelion reduces sinus inflammation and expels excess mucus (along with the allergens it carries). Indications include neck pain, low-grade spring fevers or feeling overheated, and conditions that improve with movement (including receiving bodywork) and worsen when trying to be still.

**Goldenrod (*Solidago* spp.):** A beloved ally for alleviating seasonal allergies, Goldenrod is adept at relieving congestion and sinus pain. Additional indications for Goldenrod include sore throat, eczema irritated by allergies (it makes a great salve for rashes), and asthma.

**Lemon Balm (*Melissa officinalis*):** A good tonic herb, Lemon Balm protects against overwhelm, whether that's feeling swamped by change, social situations, the effects of allergies, or whatever else is looming large in your life. Indications include itchy eyes and skin (use both internally and externally as a skin wash or steam), hay fever, and sinus headaches.

**Nettles (*Urtica dioica*):** A nutritionally dense plant ally, Nettles are a great herb for strengthening and nourishing our body. Nettles have antihistamine qualities and are traditionally described as helping to "build the blood," speaking to its iron content and overall nutritive and energizing healing qualities. Indications include general seasonal allergies, fatigue, and adrenal stress.

**Peppermint (*Mentha piperita*):** If you're feeling particularly sluggish this spring, turn to Peppermint to sweep away the remaining drowsiness of winter so you can connect with the energy of the new season. Indications include trouble breathing deeply, allergy-induced brain fog, and allergy-related pain due to inflammation.



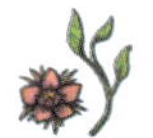

## Two Steps Forward, One Step Back: Springtime Colds & Fevers

While I've listed a few favorite spring herbs for colds and fevers, be sure to explore the winter apothecary section for a more complete list of recommendations for different types of colds, coughs, and fevers.

**Basil (*Ocimum* spp.):** Basil is one of my favorite clearing and cleansing herbs, drawing fevers out, clearing congestion, and protecting against infection. The Holy Basil (*Ocimum tenuiflorum*) variety is a useful immunomodulator and adaptogen. Indications include lethargy, brain fog, sore throat, congestion, and elevated stress.

**Cleavers (*Galium aparine*):** A wonderful daily tonic to protect against infection, Cleavers can be a great ally if a spring cold or fever arrives. Combining lymphatic, anti-inflammatory, and diaphoretic qualities, Cleavers lower fevers, clear out inflammation, and alleviate congestion. Indications include swollen lymphs, water retention, and low energy.

**Oregano (*Oregano vulgaris*):** One of the primary uses of Oregano in traditional western herbalism is for colds and flu, fighting off infection, clearing congestion, and opening up the airways. Start taking Oregano at the first sign of cold and flu to prevent or reduce symptoms. Oregano helps to break fevers and stimulate the immune system, while increasing energy during and after an illness. A key indication for Oregano is not quite getting over a cold or feeling like the immune system never "warms" up enough to properly fight off infection.

**Thyme (*Thymus vulgaris*):** As soon as Thyme returns to the garden, I begin adding a fresh sprig to my morning tea, gently staving off infection, especially of the respiratory variety. It is useful for colds and flus in general. Indications include congestion and infection, tight and high energy, and brain fog.

## Breathing Deeply: Respiratory & Lung Health

### Herbal Actions

*Anti-inflammatories, demulcents, astringents, aromatics, and expectorants*

The land breathes in different ways throughout the year, and the spring breath is a clearing and energizing one, setting us up for respiratory health for the rest of the year. Many spring herbs support general respiratory health as anti-inflammatories, but the following are a few favorite herbs for acuter respiratory support.

**Elecampane (*Inula helenium*):** A good herb for seasonal allergies and stubborn coughs of all sorts, Elecampane is especially indicated for damp coughs, painful coughs, and coughs that are worse when lying down.

**Mullein (*Verbascum thapsus*):** If you've had a long season of being sick this past winter, Mullein can be a great ally, especially if there is a lingering cough. I like combining Mullein with Elder and Peppermint for a lung-opening, immunomodulating blend. Mullein is helpful for those whose asthma is irritated by the increase in heat and allergens that spring brings. Indications include dry and spasmodic coughs, general lung weakness, and hoarseness.

**Yerba Santa (*Eriodictyon californicum*):** If you have the sort of spring allergies that cause a lot of damp and mucus, Yerba Santa might be a good ally. It's a respiratory tonic and nervine connecting us deeply to our breath and nervous system. Indications include stubborn chronic coughs and wheezing, excess mucus, and sore throat.

## The Singing Land: Herbs for the Vagus Nerve & Nervous System

### Herbal Actions

*Nervines, adaptogens, sedatives, restoratives, and analgesics*

The vagus nerve is the longest and most complex cranial nerve in the body, reaching down from the brain to the gastrointestinal tract and spreading throughout the body into our organs. It is foundational to our parasympathetic nervous system, which manages our body's homeostasis (i.e., the balance between all of our body's physiological functions) as well as the state of rest and digest. Rest and digest (or rest, digest, ground, and center) is what happens before and after a flight, fright, freeze, or fawn response and is crucial to managing our body's immune system, emotional balance, digestion, and more. The vagus nerve acts as a pathway of communication between our body systems and brain, and vice versa. Bringing the vagus nerve into a state of nourished balance is like finding your ideal harmonizing tone that connects you to the songs of life, land, and community.

**Lavender (*Lavandula* spp.):** A cooling remedy, Lavender works with the nervous system very intelligently—it stimulates a sluggish nervous system when needed, bringing clarity and focus while lifting lethargy, but can also calm an aggravated nervous system. Indications include overstimulation, agitation, nervousness, and insomnia—especially for overheated conditions such as anger and irritability.

**Lemon Balm (*Melissa officinalis*):** An herb of joy, Lemon Balm has long been prized in traditional western herbalism as a life-restoring ally. I like to think of Lemon Balm as an herb of overextension: Whether we have pushed past our boundaries through overwork, overstimulation, hyperactivity, or stress, Lemon Balm helps us to draw our energy back in and center ourselves. Indications for Lemon Balm include chronic stress, social anxiety, big life transitions, and desiring connection but struggling to show up in relationships of all kinds.

**Milky Oat (*Avena sativa*):** If I could only stock a handful of herbs in my apothecary, Milky Oat would be at the top of my list. Milky Oat is my favorite nervous system herb, and since stress is an underlying factor for most of the illnesses and symptoms I see in my practice, it is a vital and beloved plant ally of mine. Milky Oat is a nervous system trophorestorative, making it an ideal plant ally for most any vagus nerve needs. Indications include general fatigue, loss of hope and inspiration, stress and anxiety, trouble sleeping, and a general feeling of discombobulation in the body.

**Rose (*Rosa* spp.):** Rose is an ancient, ancestral plant ally, having watched us evolve as a species, so what better herb to turn to when tending the central pathways of communication and experience of our bodies. In addition to being an excellent overall vagus nerve tonic, Rose is indicated for any sort of ancestral work, including exploring and healing intergenerational trauma and setting boundaries.

**Skullcap (*Scutellaria lateriflora*):** A powerful nervine, Skullcap restores strength to an overwhelmed nervous system, relieving spasms and nerve pain and cultivating calm. Indications include difficulty resting or focusing because of constant mental chatter, insomnia, and general hyperactivity.

## Arriving Earthside: Herbs to Support Pregnancy, Birth & Postpartum

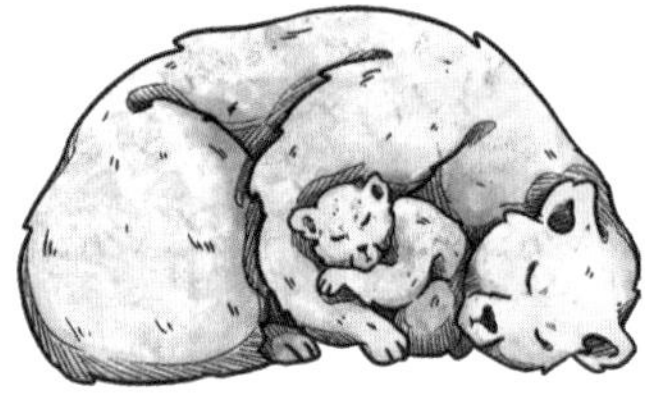

### *Herbal Actions*

*Uterine tonics, nervines, analgesics, anti-inflammatory, and antihemorrhagic*

Working with herbs to support pregnant, birthing, and postpartum people is a specialty, and one that deserves time, practice, and experience, but there are a few general recommendations I can make about this part of the life cycle so deeply tied to the land in spring. Many of these herbs can also be used in either plant or flower essence form for folks exploring the energetic process of being fertile with an idea and bringing a project into the world. While you should always consult your midwife, herbalist, and/or medical practitioner before taking herbs during pregnancy, birth, and postpartum, the following are generally considered safe.

**Chamomile (*Matricaria chamomilla*):** If you're experiencing insomnia during pregnancy and beyond, Chamomile can be a great ally. Chamomile is also beneficial for the emotional ups and downs of postpartum, as well as for supporting digestion throughout this time.

**Lemon Balm (*Melissa officinalis*):** A gentle herb, Lemon Balm alleviates stress and anxiety, supports rest, and can help folks connect to the joyful aspects of the pregnancy and postpartum experience.

**Nettles (*Urtica dioica*):** During pregnancy, Nettles act as a wonderful daily multivitamin for the parent and growing fetus. It is useful throughout postpartum, too, internally, for rebuilding strength and externally for perineal repair. Nettles have an amphoteric effect on the milk supply—increasing milk if there is too little or reducing it if there is too much.

## The Childhood of the Year: Herbs for Children

### *Herbal Actions*

*Nervines, immunomodulators, analgesics, and vulneraries*

As a season traditionally associated with childhood, springtime can be a beautiful period to explore plant life with children as well as create herbal remedies for the little ones in your life. Many herbs that show up in spring are effective yet gentle remedies for common childhood ailments, but here are a few favorites. These herbs can also be used in either plant form or as a flower essence for inner child work and healing.

**Calendula (*Calendula officinalis*):** I make a Calendula salve, my absolute favorite topical treatment for little ones, each year for rashes, massages to get lymph nodes working in cases of illness, and all variety of wound care, including insect bites, bruises, scrapes, burns, and general inflammation. Calendula is easy to grow, and little ones can participate in picking the bright flowers to make into an herbal oil to be used as is or blended into a salve.

**Catnip (*Nepeta cataria*):** A great herb for calming and soothing agitated and nervous little ones. Catnip can also be added to blends for colds, flu, and coughs and makes a great component in herbal baths. Indications for Catnip include insomnia caused by anxiety and nightmares, dry skin and overheating, as well as teething pain.

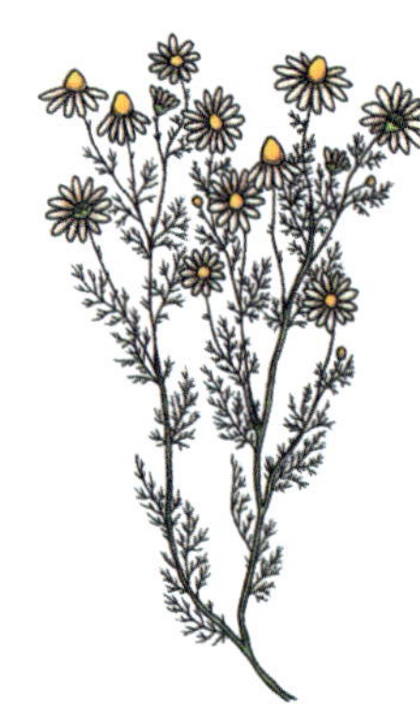

**Chamomile (*Matricaria chamomilla*):** Chamomile is one of my favorite herbs for all varieties of childhood complaints, from upset stomach, nervousness, cold and flu to invoking calm in the mind and body. It's a classic remedy for the colicky and sensitive child whose emotional disturbances and overstimulation are felt through their stomachs. Chamomile kids often complain of an upset stomach when their internal or external environment feels unsteady. Additional indications for Chamomile include increased sensitivity to pain, using anger as a shield (resulting in trapped heat), and restlessness.

**Elder (*Sambucus nigra*):** Elderberry syrup is a beloved remedy in my apothecary, gentle enough for all ages and protective against viruses and infections. Elderberry clears congested passageways and acts as an immunomodulator, making it a good choice to take over an extended period of cold and flu season. Indications for Elder include reddishness, dryness, and irritability, as well as poor circulation and low immunity (as when your kid seems to catch every cold that comes their way).

**Lemon Balm (*Melissa officinalis*):** This is one of my favorite remedies for littles ones with a cold or flu. For feverish children consider combining Lemon Balm with Elderflower and Elderberry, Chamomile, and Peppermint. Alternatively, use as a bath for children unable or resistant to taking tea. Lemon Balm can be drunk as a tea before bed to alleviate nightmares and is good for children who are prone to anxiety about school, exams, and performances. Indications for Lemon Balm include nervousness and agitation, helping children deal with feelings of disappointment, grief, and general anxiety.

**Peppermint (*Mentha piperita*):** Another lovely and pleasant-tasting herb, Peppermint can be added to blends for cold and flu, respiratory inflammation, allergies, and indigestion. With its distinctive scent and flavor, Peppermint is an herb kids can learn to identify quickly, helping them feel connected to the world of plants. Indications for Peppermint include nausea (including travel sickness), headaches, indigestion, and lack of focus.

**The Community Clinic in Spring**

*Anti-inflammatory and antihistamine teas for seasonal allergies*

*Soothing anti-itch balms for skin transitioning from winter to spring and general seasonal allergies*

*Clearing circulatory tonics for lymph health*

*Calming hydrosols for the skin and energy field*

*Relaxing teas for the nervous system*

*Respiratory tonics to support airways and restorative breathwork*

*Nutrient-rich teas to rebuild strength after winter*

# Spring Recipes & Rituals

These three recipes support the seasons of the land of your body, helping to energize, soothe, and nourish our inner landscape. Formulated as teas, they can also be made into extracts; see the Folk Remedy-Making Guide for brewing instructions.

## Energizing Spring Tea

If we are feeling ready to meet the new season ahead but need extra help with the transition, an energizing seasonal blend can be useful. Herbs like bitters, circulatory tonics, and energizing nervines can align us with the energy of spring. An energizing blend is less about being stimulating and more about supporting the body in ways that allows energy to flow freely.

2 parts Lemon Balm (*Melissa officinalis*)
1 part Peppermint (*Mentha piperita*)
½ part Dandelion Leaf & Flower (*Taraxacum officinale*)

## Soothing Spring Tea

Sometimes we need to calm, ground, and settle energy that feels frayed, out of sorts, and/or overwhelming. While we might strive to feel at one with every season of the year and of our lives, the truth is sometimes a season can be hard and we struggle to feel resonance with the land. For a soothing spring blend I recommend relaxing nervines and heart tonics to help us settle. Adaptogens are a useful addition when recovering from a period of heightened stress.

3 parts Holy Basil (*Ocimum tenuiflorum*)
1 part Skullcap *(Scutellaria lateriflora)*
½ part Rose *(Rosa spp.)*

## Nourishing Spring Tea

A nourishing blend incorporates nutritive and tonic herbs that work with the energy of the season to help our inner landscape flourish. I recommend combining one or more of your favorite tonic herbs that can be taken over an extended period of time (ideally the full season) alongside herbs that are in season. Nourishing blends are especially appropriate for rebuilding energy reserves after a period of illness, calling ourselves home to the land, and supporting cycles of realigning and remembering what it is we feel called to do in our life.

1 part Nettles (*Urtica dioica*)
1 part Milky Oat (*Avena sativa*)
1 part Chamomile (*Matricaria chamomilla*)

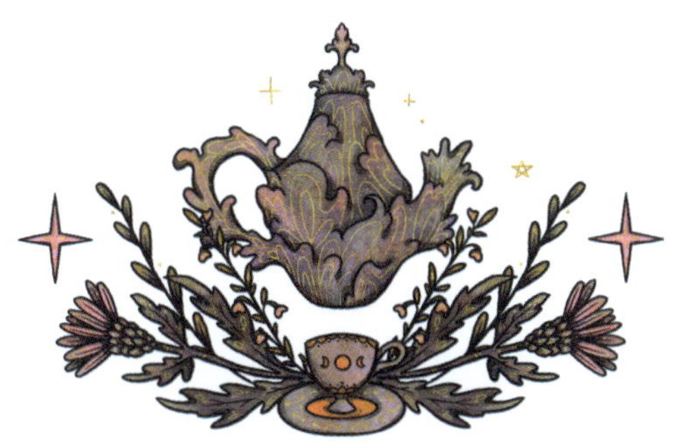

## The Witch's Ladder of Light Ritual

Witch's ladders are an old form of folk magick where items such as feathers are knotted or braided into a cord, often to bring about healing by "tying up" and removing illness from someone. I love working with witch's ladders during the bright and windy times of year like spring as they are a beautiful form of air magick. They are also a sort of magick that can help us along paths of grief, reminding us of simple pleasures and the promise of a gentler future. On a bright spring day, we can create a witch's ladder that ties up a bit of sunlight to use as a guiding torch to bring with us throughout the year.

**You will need:**

A length of cord, yarn, or rope
Eight fresh or dried herb stalks, feathers, or charms of your choosing
A bell

On a bright spring day, lay your objects in a sunny spot, preferably outside but beside a sunny window will do, too. You can use feathers for your witch's ladder, connecting to the lineage of witchfolk gone before; dried or fresh herb stalks; or charms or small beads that represent hopeful and steadying energy to you (e.g., symbols of a holy one you work with or citrine beads and Calendula flowers for their bright, solar quality).

Begin by blessing each of your chosen objects, holding them one by one to the sunlight, saying each time:

*Every one a home for light*
*to shine in the dark*
*as hope becomes bright*

Hold up the cord to the sunlight and bless it by saying:

*A path of light*
*that holds the sun*
*guide me when*
*all seems undone*

Next, begin knotting or braiding in your chosen objects one by one, and as you work, visualize the light of spring being gathered up and stored in each object and held in place by your knot or braid. As you incorporate an object, name the hope it carries, such as "joy" or "peace" or something more specific to your experience such as "the feeling of waking up from a beautiful dream."

Add the bell last, saying:

*As I ring*
*the light sings*


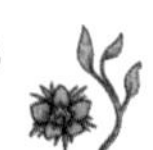

Once all your chosen objects have been attached, bless your witch's ladder of light by holding it up to the sun and saying

*Beauty of spring*
*hope of light—*
*I carry you with me*
*every day, every night!*
*So mote it be!*

## Calling in the Future Community Ritual

Spring's brightening weather carries in the winds of change, clearing out stagnant energy and supporting us in envisioning futures of a more just and more kind world. Holding a ritual with your community—whether a coven, organizing committee, or family circle—where you name and call in the visions of a future you want to bring about can be a powerful act of magick.

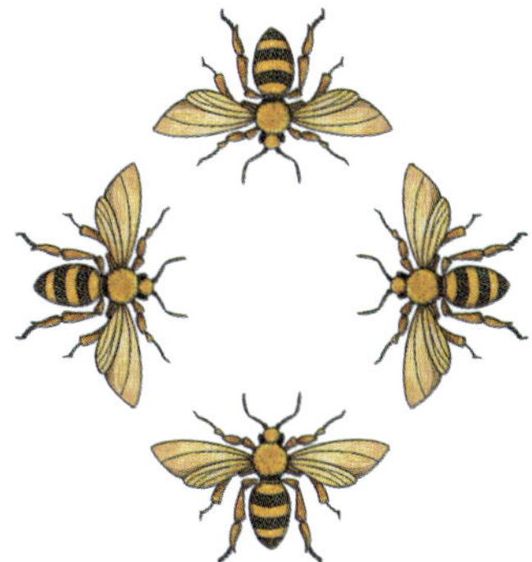

The power of a community imagining its future into being was a lesson I was fortunate enough to learn early in my organizing days, and it has shaped my work ever since. Envisioning what a future aligned with values of compassion and healing reciprocity might look like, instead of only focusing on the easy-to-name things that we *don't* want in our futures, takes effort but is transformative. Depending on your community culture, you can add as much ritual and symbolism as you want to the following steps, but the heart of the rite is taking a moment to dwell together with the future you're calling in.

**You will need:**

Thyme
Rose
Lemon Balm tea or herbs meaningful to your community

Begin by taking time to talk together about the future you're trying to bring in. A community clinic might envision what their community would look like if they had all the resources they need and culturally competent, evidence-based care was abundantly available. Or an abolitionist community might discuss what a vibrant local economy would look like, from local businesses to urban farms to community colleges, when their youth aren't entrapped in prison systems but free to pursue their life's callings. A coven might envision what it would feel like to have a safe space to practice outside, while a family might dream of a future when they take regular time off together and how they might be transformed by the results of traveling to places they've always dreamed of. You're not trying to predict the future and this is not a planning meeting where you're figuring out logistics—this is solely a visioning exercise where you imagine and spend time in a desired future.

To begin, one or more people should be designated as the facilitators to keep the ritual flowing. I've suggested things to say, but please adapt any and all of it to make sense for your community. Follow the emotional current—it can stretch from the serious to the laughter-rich, the profound to the very mundane—so adapt as needed.

When you're ready, gather in a circle. While I envision a space where herbs can be used to draw circles on the ground, you can perform the same ritual gestures by placing herbs on a small plate or tray in the middle of those gathered and energetically moving in the circles.

To begin, the ritual facilitator lets everyone know that it's time to visit the future together, to call these visions into the present. For groups that work with trance techniques or guided meditations, you can incorporate some of that here to help folks move into a deeper ritual space.

With Thyme, create a circle in the center of those gathered, large enough for someone to move into and either stand or sit. Thyme helps us to move backward and forward through time and space; we'll be using it to call the future in.

The facilitator speaks:

*The time is now! Who visits us from the future?*

Now is when an individual from the community moves forward into the circle of Thyme and acts out who they are or an archetype of this called-in future. A community clinic member, for example, might step forward and joyfully share how wonderful it is to finally be in a fully accessible space all abilities can visit! And there's a garden where they can grow their own herbs!

Once the community member is done sharing, the facilitator steps forward and offers them some Rose petals, instructing them to sprinkle the petals as they leave the circle of Thyme and go back to their spot in the wider circle. Rose is an herb of the time between and gateways, pulling the envisioned future toward the present.

One by one community members move into the circle of Thyme, share their vision, and make a path of Rose petals as they leave. Once everyone who wants to share has spoken, the facilitator speaks again:

*We call in the time we already know is coming*
*We call in what we need and know will arrive*
*We call in—*

Community members name aloud the resources required to bring the future they've all just witnessed. Shout it out! Whisper it intensely! Raise energy in any way your community knows how. Finally, the facilitator leads everyone in grounding the energy of the ritual, encouraging folks by saying this or something similar:

*Yes, it's here, we've called it in! Blessed be!*

Let folks move around, circle dance, stop and sing if they feel called. Once the energy has peaked and ebbed, it's time to share Lemon Balm tea to fully integrate and harmonize the community vision with everyone gathered.

## The Dreamer's Oracle

Drawing upon spring's energy, we can use our oracle of belonging to explore how our dreams are appearing in our inner landscape and connect with plant allies to support our dream's healing message.

Choose three plant allies, whether the actual herb or a symbol of the plant ally:

> one to represent your dream
> one to represent your dreaming self
> one to represent your waking self

Prepare your space, making a spring-inspired tea if you like, and lay your oracle of belonging out before you. Ground, center, and speak any divining charms you wish. When ready, take up your herbs or objects, close your eyes, and either toss or place them at random on the oracle map. For spring, I like to close my eyes and slowly spiral my hand above the oracle, in a deosil motion, until I intuitively feel the spot where I should place my herb or object.

Where the dream herb or object lands tells you about what area of your inner landscape this dream has been generated from or is speaking most directly to. The placement of the dreaming self object represents the meaning of the dream. The waking self's placement represents the way the dream is showing up in your present, waking life.

Let's say that the dream object lands in the oracle area representing your past, speaking to the dream being tied up to old energy you've been carrying around. The dreaming self object may land on the space representing your heart-self, suggesting this dream's meaning is tied up with the feelings of love, perhaps rejection, or some ongoing healing of a broken heart. Finally, the waking self marker lands in the area of air and communication in your chart, possibly suggesting something needs to be said about this issue of the heart for healing to take place.

From the oracle you might feel inspired to work with plant allies to integrate the dream's healing message into your life, choosing one to three herbs to represent the healing energy of the dream, the part of you that dreamed it, and your waking self's physical needs.


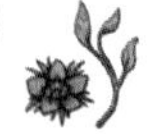

## The New Moon

Within the astrological roots of traditional western herbalism, the new moon is a time of hot and moist herbs, corresponding to the damp and increasing warmth spring brings. While spring arrives with the strongest current of fresh beginnings, momentum, and tenderhearted possibility, each month the new moon carries this same energy that we can connect to throughout the year.

In my own lunar practice, I enjoy harvesting plants and making remedies that correspond to the energies of release (the scythe-shaped new moon helps us to cut away unwanted energy and attachments) and increasing vitality, including restorative nervous system tonics, stress relief blends, and recipes that warm up the inner digestive fire.

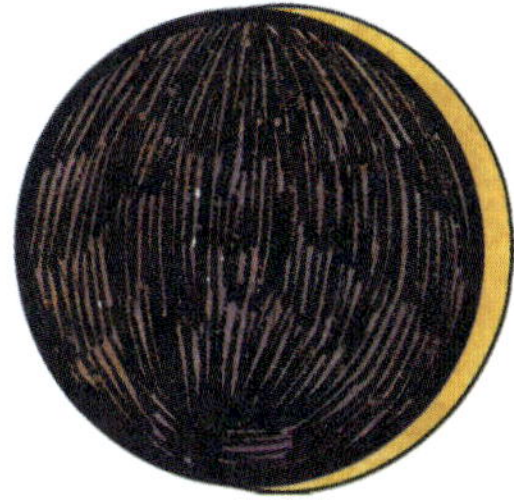

### *New Moon Remedy Blessing*

To be said over remedies while making them, during their brewing process, and/or before administering them:

*By the light of the new moon*
*untangle and unbind*
*clear the path of healing*
*make it easy to find*

*as moonlight grows*
*so does the remedy*
*land, body, heart*
*all in serenity*

*blessed be*

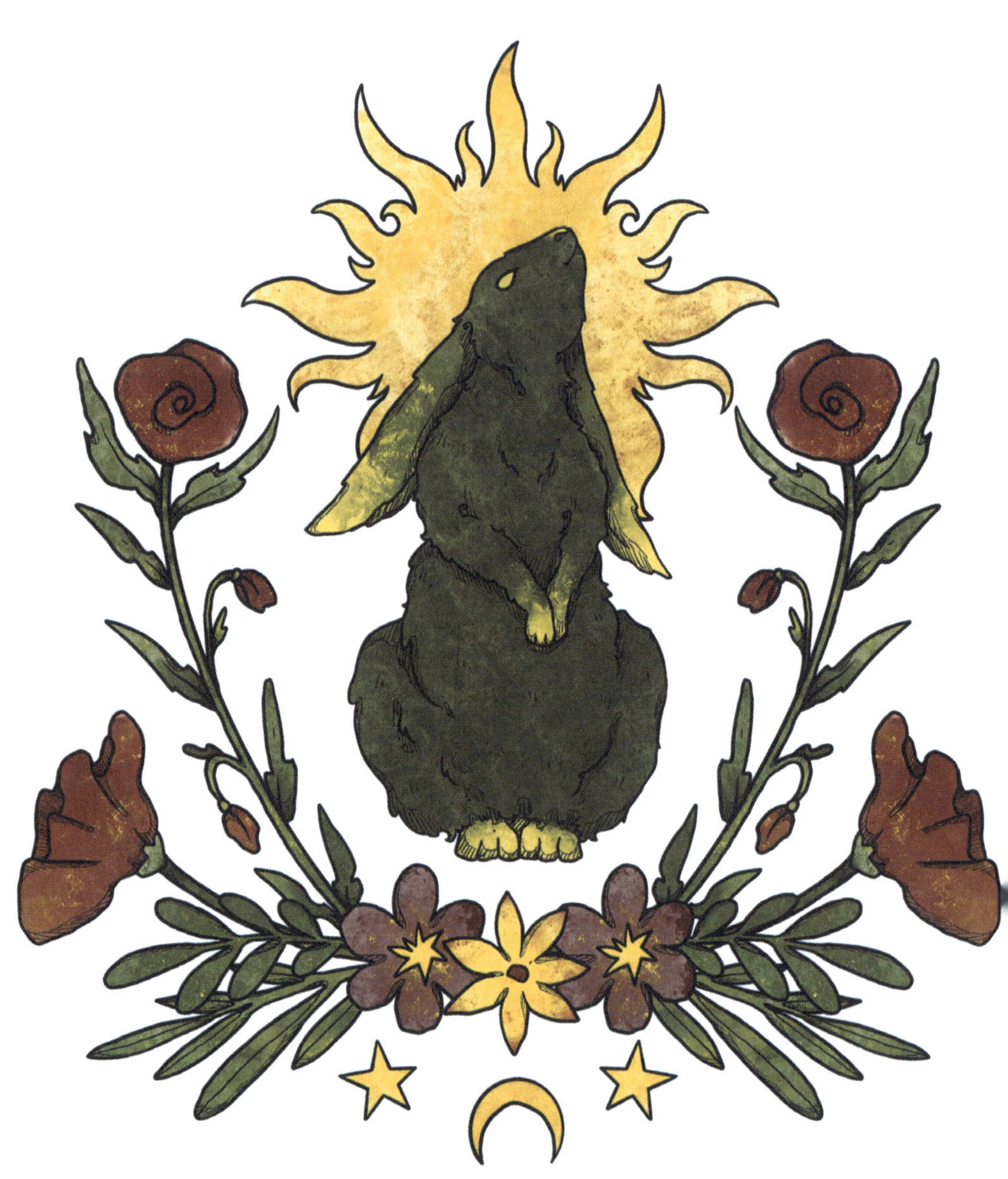

# Summer

Summer comes rushing in, urged on by the energetic sweep of spring, bringing heat and dryness to the land. Our land-bodies move from spring's quick dance of growth to the settling maturation of summer, pulling us from the *what might be* of spring into the *what is right now* of summer. We are in the season of the long sun, tucked in between the rush of spring and the long hours of fall harvest, when energy steadies and lengthens, making plenty of time for community gatherings, celebrating commitments and unions, and storytelling that inspires change. The land in summer buzzes with life and light, granting us the gift of time-making, when we can stretch out into new and remembered spaces, intermingled with bonfire and starlight.

The myths of summer are many, from tree kings engaging in friendly competition to humans tumbling into the enchanted lands of Good Folk. In summer, time seems to slow and spaces seem to take on a languid, otherworldly glow. Many of summer's tales revolve around the experience of time changing: from the last of winter giving way to the power of summer to humans returning from one night's revelry in the otherworld to find years have passed in their own. In agricultural societies where summer was less busy compared to planting and harvesting seasons, community gatherings were easier to host where stories and news of the year could be exchanged, with the longer days also making it easier to travel greater distances.

Carried by stories and community connections from the tender momentum of spring, we grow into the sturdier, braver, and hopefully a little bit wiser season of summer. The long days provide space to test out and develop new skills, revisit old ones, and explore our spring dreams with summer theories. We help our summer selves bloom by turning to heart tonics, remedies supporting our gut flora and digestive fire, nourishing skin treatments, and fertility aids of both the physical and creative varieties.

In traditional western herbalism, summer is a time of air meeting fire, supporting a long, hot season of growth, a period of archetypal youth (i.e., teenagers and young adults), the energy of the compass direction south (or north in the Southern Hemisphere), and the abundance of the waxing quarter moon. Through fire, we physically and energetically extend our awareness with movement, seeking the wisdom gained only through connecting with others and letting ourselves be moved by and through the land as our inner fire calls us to.

During these long, hot days, our summer selves seek out places, people, systems, and philosophies that help us grow what it is that inspired us most during the spring. We find ourselves drawn outdoors to the shelter of shade and stretching toward communion with the land and our communities, and just as the land around us grows and shifts in interesting ways during summer, so can we. Through our play and explorations, the season of abundance strengthens us with the charm of gratitude, when we realize summer's youthful vigor is only possible through the vulnerable work of the land and our communities throughout the rest of the year. With so much energy in the air, hot and rising, we must be wary of going too hard for too long, turning instead to the land and our plant allies to help us discern the practices needed to store some of this energy to draw upon later during the colder months of the year.

What shape will the tenderness of spring take when held by the sheltering warmth and light of summer?

**Sweet Spring, Bright Summer Breathwork**

*Find a comfortable position, perhaps under the easy light of the rising or setting sun, and take a few centering breaths. Either close your eyes or let the edges of your vision soften as you breathe in to a count of four (or a count that feels most comfortable for you), visualizing summer's light filling you up. Hold your breath for a count of four, then exhale for a count of four, letting summer's light flow easily around you. Breathe in again for a count of four and continue in this pattern of breathing for at least nine rounds. As you do this breathwork, you can adjust the length of your count up or down as you need. As you continue to breathe in this steady pattern, imagine your energy gently and comfortably extending outward, creating a strengthening aura of summer light around you.*


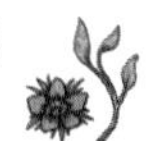

## The Gifts of Summer

### *Gratitude*

Summer is here—the starkness of winter is a distant memory, the busyness of autumn not yet arrived, and the tender life of spring grown into something a little steadier, more confident, more robust. It can be easy to feel grateful during the long, languid days of summer when life and time are abundant. Summer can enchant us with its song of plenty, and one of its strongest rhythms is gratitude. Gratitude is a powerful practice of observation, community-building, and land-reconnection, helping us recognize what makes us glad-hearted. The early plants of spring have blossomed into the steady growth of summer, giving back to the soil as they root deeper into the earth, yet still full of promise for the harvest ahead. When we meet summer in our own inner landscapes, we feel more confident in who we are and the gifts we bring to our lives and communities.

When I think of gratitude, I think of summer bonfires lighting up across the land, from backyards to hilltops, between sacred stones and shorelines, in hearths and in hearts. Bonfires make me think of all the ways gratitude and listening to what other folks are grateful for can help us become generous of heart and action. Starting from at least sixty thousand years ago during the Old Stone Age, our ancestors have been working with plants as medicine. It was during this same period that we also found some of the earliest examples of art, from sculptures like the Venus of Willendorf to cave paintings of animals, geometric shapes for decoration or to mark maps and calendars, and generations of stamped and stenciled handprints. Around ancient cookfires, stories were shared, advice given, food passed, and something created between people that wouldn't exist without the exchange of ideas and knowledge. My gratitude for these ancient peoples and their observations of the world that led to the development of traditions like herbal and modern medicine can sometimes feel overwhelming—what a profound lineage we are all born from.

I am grateful, too, for the land that has provided for generations and to all of our nonhuman kin, knowing that there were many moments when our ancient ancestors observed how animals interacted with plants in order to understand their uses. It is incredible what knowledge has survived, shared first by storytelling and in the libraries of cave art. Cultivating a gratitude practice is a powerful act of ancestral healing, and it can help to work with plants that have been on our planet for millennia, such as Rose (*Rosa* spp.) and Ginkgo (*Ginkgo biloba*), when trying to connect with our long human legacy.

I was first introduced to the practice of gratitude as a teenager, reading in one of my books on magick about how gratitude was recognizing the abundance that already existed in your life in order to grow more of it.[6] Every evening before bed I would link paper clips, each representing something I was grateful for that day. These long lengths of little metal clips helped me notice and hold in my hands—and begin to feel in my body—those things that held me in my life, softening the shoulders of teenage angst, giving myself some perspective, and eventually leading me to explore the world of class, access, and the politics of labor throughout my youth and young adulthood. Gratitude is a skill that can be developed, giving people of all ages, but especially younger ones, the space to get to know themselves as individuals while recognizing cohesive family and community structures for them to thrive in as interconnected and beloved members of a greater whole.

For too many of us, though, the closest we got to a gratitude practice was through being instructed (mostly by older folks in positions of authority) to be grateful for whatever it was they provided. Being "grateful" in these circumstances was a way to force conformity rather than an invitation to an actual connection. In its more pernicious form, demands for gratitude from those around us can take on an air of toxic positivity or be a thin excuse for abusive situations. Untangling the "you should be grateful" pattern is an important part of developing a true embodied gratitude that protects us from developing a hostility toward sharing the abundance of our ocean planet. A gratitude practice should be an invitation to expansiveness and a way for the land of our bodies to experience the vital wellspring of summer's long-lasting hope.

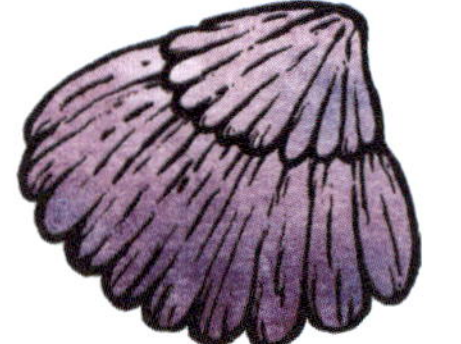

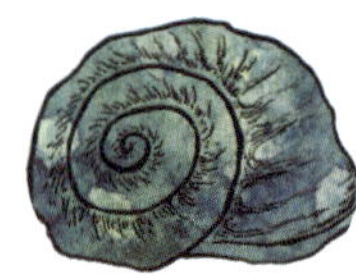

Sometimes, the idea of a gratitude practice feels less like a gentle summer stroll and closer to feeling exposed under the scorching midday sun. Gratitude can be a challenging practice because it is an exercise in observation, recognition, and naming, leading us to consider our inner and outer worlds with more nuance, recognize what feels abundant and lacking in our life, and name why that is. For folks just starting to explore the dynamics of access and oppression, institutional and interpersonal systems of power, and our many identities—all of which are necessary for creating an enduring healing practice—I encourage developing a gratitude practice because it can be all too easy to get lost in an ocean of guilt, despair, and/or shame when we don't have sight of the shoreline. And all these brave explorations, these complex experiences of inheritance and lived experience, and these generations of trauma intermingled with generations of wisdom can be a lot to hold. Even though our ancient ancestors passed down wisdom, not everything old is good, so traditions need to be renewed through cyclical and collective reexamination. Plant allies like Rose (*Rosa* spp.), Milky Oat (*Avena sativa*), Hawthorn (*Crataegus monogyna*), and Motherwort (*Leonurus cardiaca*) can help us navigate our experiences and refine our discernment while soothing our heart and nervous system.

Gratitude is our sightline, reminding us why we get into the work of restorative healing. With all of its mystery and uncomfortable vulnerability, it is through gratitude that we remember why we are doing all this. Looking out over the land in summer, it can be easy to spot abundance, and just like in the cold depths of winter, under the shadeless heat of summer we can easily identify any lack. Summer is a time of pausing and planning. We can pinpoint where resources are lacking, what needs to be built for the dark of the year, and move together in a spirit of gratitude that helps us to see what skills we already have, while carrying the stories of our ancestors alongside the bold, unhindered wisdom of our youthful descendants. What gratitude in your life helps you keep sight of the shoreline and your safe harbors?

I know so many folks called to the path of healing and restorative justice because of their deep gratitude for the people, places, and nonhuman kin who were there at their most vulnerable moments. Gratitude is hope in action and the foundation of reciprocal relationships, guiding us through some of our most challenging conversations. In my own practice, the opportunities for gratitude are endless! I'm grateful for the trees and hedges that sheltered me as a kid, the people who've done this work before me, who taught me how to listen, speak my heart, and spot places for connection. I'm grateful for those who've shown up in my consultations and classrooms asking for help and seeking knowledge and those who have made space for me to show up in all my unsteadiness and for being shown when I need to get out of the summer's glare and into summer's shade. In my practice of gratitude I try to answer the question, *What are the ways that I am showing reverence and gratefulness to the land, the people, and nonhuman kin who I am interconnected with?*

Physically, at the end of spring and beginning of summer, we might need to rebuild our energy after a season of allergens has left us depleted and run-down. Many summer herbs are not only nutrient-dense but reenergizing for our body systems, helping us store vital energy for the rest of the year. Incorporating, as well as making remedies of, nutritive nervines, cardiotonics, and adaptogens can help us flow through summer with ease as well as protect us against illness during colder months.

## *Shelter*

Every season I look for shelter. I find the shelter of hope in spring and then summer's shelter of shade and languid time, while autumn brings the shelter of the harvest table and winter offers the shseleter of hearth and good company. Existing between spring's planting season and the harvest of autumn, summer is a time of shelter-making, of house-building and barn-raising, circle dances, community meetings, project expansions, and plenty of time gathered on city blocks and public parks for cookouts and parties.

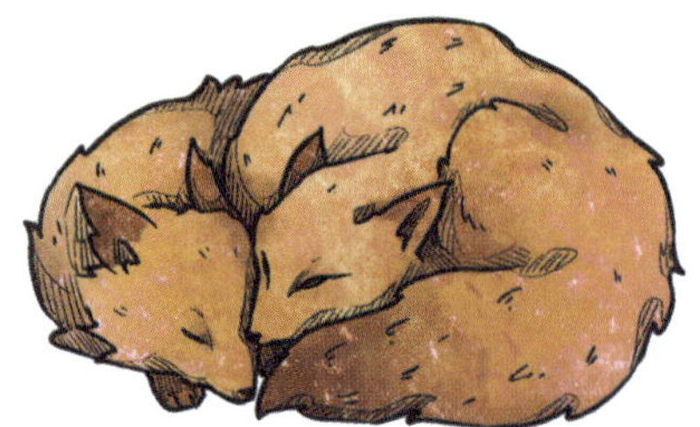

It is through sitting with the practice of gratitude and being part of communities and relationships doing healing work that I've come to appreciate how intrinsically gratitude and shelter are tied together. It's not unusual for our gratitude practices to lead us to recognize how we've been sheltered—whether the physical shelter of a safe home, the emotional shelter of an attentive parent or compassionate partner(s), or the shelter of a spiritual practice that helps us find the meaning in our life. It's no surprise then, that through figuring out what we are grateful for, we learn what it is we want to shelter and protect. Everyone can find rituals of sheltering among their ancestral lines, and there are many examples of ancient summer—and, more generally, fire—festivals where protective energy is called in and baneful energy driven out. Just as there are many ways to express gratitude in our lives, there are many ways to create shelter for the people, places, items, and ideas we want to protect. Looking around the land I live with, I can find so many examples of shelter, like the towering Oaks that have provided generations of shelter through shade and homes within their branches, through food and dyestuff, medicines, and building materials for a variety of species. Watching the land in summer we can learn to spot the interconnected strands of shelter and how to participate in their systems throughout all seasons of the year and our lives.

One way I offer shelter to the land and kin I live with is to allow for lots of wild edges and deep layers of shade in our garden space. Not only is the texture of varied layers and variety of plant and tree life healing to look at and be around, but it is an effective way to create habitat for all kinds of animals, insects, and spirits of the land. There is more opportunity for rainwater to find its way into the soil instead of down the sewers, more plant and tree fall to create layered, nutrient-rich dirt, and greater chance for practical shelter to be found throughout the seasons. As we learn to work with the land around us from a perspective of kinship and shelter, reverence and reciprocity, we can turn these practices inward for our own landed bodies. My inner sky surrounds me like our planet's sheltering ozone, helping me create a porous and protective barrier around myself. When kindness, like rainfall, comes my way, I want to be able to soak it up so it helps me grow. I try to let myself be nourished by a variety of sources, opening to a diversity of nutrients for my inner earth instead of trying to narrowly force myself to grow through one type of relationship, expectation, experience, or belief.

As we practice gratitude and seek out shelter, there are times we'll find ourselves traveling through the gates of our inner and collective underworlds, through hidden constellations of mycelium, past bones and stones, and beyond crystal caverns. Through our journeys, we leave behind what we fear we don't have enough of, what we're afraid might be taken from us, what we believe we need to hoard or hide, and we return to the surface, like a flower emerging from bud into full bloom, with our gratitude humming within us. To avoid shelter, and any underworld journeys it may call us to, is to avoid connection. Humans have sheltered in trees and caves, using what land and kin provided in the form of plant, bone, skin, and stone to then start building and designing places to live. But we have also sheltered each other through shared values and alliances, familial and tribal ties, in ways that not only reshaped *us* as a species, but also our nonhuman kin like dogs, cows, and horses, as well as the land. We have to guard against the baneful belief that another person's shelter threatens our own, that those without shelter are somehow less deserving of it, or that being and feeling sheltered are a privilege not a right. As you practice in the world, it can be helpful to notice the way your healing work shelters and how you might extend or refine that sheltering energy to be more inclusive, kind, and sustainable to yourself and the planet. Gratitude shelters through the generations, and so we, like our ancestors before us, are called to participate in this long weaving of wisdom, braiding summer light for our descendants to carry with them into the future.

As the land blooms, shaded by mature trees and sheltered by a sky blue cradle, summer offers sturdy and nutrient-rich plants to strengthen our body systems and build up our energy. Nutritive plants like Nettles (*Urtica dioica*), Dandelion (*Taraxacum officinale*), Milky Oat (*Avena sativa*), and Red Clover (*Trifolium pratense*) help us bring the spring body into summer, maturing our vitality while providing nutrients to support our longevity. When sitting with clients, I look for signs of too much exposure and the need for more sheltering energy. A client recovering from heartbreak, for example, may feel like their heart is raw and tender, leading to anxiety and mild palpitations related to


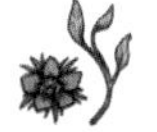

stress. Offering a cardiotonic like Hawthorn (*Crataegus monogyna*), which not only alleviates stress and regulates cardiac function, but also acts as a protective barrier for the energetic heart, creates space for them to feel sheltered as they recover. We can also carry the sheltering strength of summer with us throughout every season, drawing on summer's nutritive remedies during the leaner times of year.

All my herbal consultations involve some level of sheltering practice, helping folks find sanctuary in their lives. There is the practical work of introducing them to whole plant remedies for a healing shelter and relief from suffering in their life. Yet a lot of sheltering work is simply reflecting back to folks the practices they already have in place and that we can build upon to help them feel even better (e.g., they'll now have an herbal tea in addition to their lovely morning coffee) as well as presenting to them ways of connecting to the stories of their body with plant allies. Our stories can shelter us if we let them and if we let ourselves sit around our inner campfire and open up to the personal myths and tales we carry within us. We are being vulnerable when we say something is wrong and ask for help, when we seek out practitioners and wisdom keepers, trained and skilled professionals who are compassionate, inclusive, and culturally competent, who set out to create a supportive space for us to heal in. So I try to provide folks with resources to kindle hope—to illuminate their path, follow bonfires toward community, and learn how to light their own.

A shelter is a boundary, containing and keeping out certain experiences while simultaneously inviting in others. It helps us navigate our experiences with the predominant energy of summer—the element of fire. Fire is transformative, molten and volcanic, contained within tiny sparks and buried embers, destroying and creating with its intensity. Within Western esoteric tradition fire is the element of the heart, referring to both the energetic heart of feeling and emotional intelligence, connection, and spiritual subtlety, as well as the physical heart muscle. For our species and many mammals, without a beating heart and the animating heat of fire, there is no life. Through fire and the adventures of the heart, we learn what it is to be sheltered by heat, to be burned, to be creative, to be overcome with the fierceness of feeling, and what boundaries we need in order to feel supported and safe. In traditional western herbalism, the seats of fire in the body include the heart, gallbladder, and external reproductive organs, and fire is used as Heat and Dryness in the body and environment to bring about healing. Herbs like Nettles (*Urtica dioica*), Angelica (*Angelica archangelica*), Basil (*Ocimum* spp.), Rosemary (*Salvia rosmarinus*), and St. Joan's Wort (*Hypericum perforatum*) all possess strong fire energy, supporting the fire of our land-body.

Connecting with and supporting our heart are beautiful ways of working with the elemental energy of fire that summer brings as well as the wisdom of gratitude and practice of shelter. The energy of fire brings creativity and expansiveness, which supports our ability to experience gratitude and shelter in our lives, but when we are struggling to process fire energy, we can feel burned-out, unable to keep our energy balanced (either falling into lethargy or hyperactivity), angry and irritated (our gallbladder overworked), and uncomfortably sensitive to our inner and outer environments. Creative pursuits (including art therapy), quiet and centering activities (when there is too much fire), or exciting and energizing activities (for too little fire), as well as paying attention to your heart's desires, can help you connect to your inner fire. Some of my favorite heart-nourishing activities include these:

- Breathwork with a heart-opening focus
- Energizing movement that builds up a sweat
- Having a date with yourself and/or loved ones where you bring a creative pursuit to work on
- Dancing and making music
- Visioning practices and rituals
- Working with flowers and leaves nourishing to the heart like Hawthorn (*Crataegus monogyna*) and Rose (*Rosa* spp.), as well as blood-building tonics like Nettles (*Urtica dioica*)


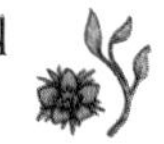

## Summer Inquiry

*What is my summer story?*

*What does summer feel, look, smell, and taste like in my body?*

*What does summer feel, look, smell, and taste like in the land around me?*

*Where am I feeling gratitude in my life and body?*

*Where do I find expressions of gratitude in the land and in my communities?*

*Where is my gratitude guiding me?*

*What kind of shelter did I receive in my youth? What was nourishing? What was lacking?*

*How do I feel sheltered in my current life?*

*How do I help to shelter others?*

## Herbs for the Summer Body

Within traditional western herbalism, summer is a time of dry air coming together with the heat of fire, when spring's softness transforms into summer's radiance. Throughout the land, growth is abundant; the high water levels of spring slowly decrease through the long days of heat and evaporation, and increased dryness can create a season of steady growth. Summer's dryness completes what was started in spring, moving the energy up from the land toward the energetic peak of the summer solstice. Within our apothecaries we can support the energy of summer by having plenty of cooling remedies on hand, lots of nervines that soothe the nervous system, digestive bitters that nourish the liver and gallbladder, strengthening blood and circulatory herbs, expansive heart tonics, and adaptogens that tap into the fire and heat of the season, gathering up summer's light for the rest of the year.

During summer, the traditional western energetics of Heat and Dryness are on the rise, and we need to be mindful of too much of either creating an inhospitable environment for healing energy to be stored and nourished. Excess Heat can generate excess energy, showing up as restlessness, sleep issues, and an increasing intensity in relationships of all kinds. Excess Heat can create issues with the immune system and inflammation, fibromyalgia, hyper-issues (e.g., hyperthyroidism, hypersensitivity, hyperactivity), and insomnia. Anger, boredom, nervousness, and restlessness are also key indicators of excess Heat. The balancing of summer energy so that it doesn't become too overheated or too subdued through too much artificial coldness (such as too much time spent in air-conditioned buildings) can be aided by tending to our internal digestive fires with heat-balancing herbal bitters like Dandelion (*Taraxacum officinale*), Chamomile (*Matricaria chamomilla*), and Peppermint (*Mentha piperita*).

As the moisture of spring is dispersed in summer, we need to be mindful of too much Dryness creating feelings of rawness and overwhelm, leading to slow recovery from illness and any sort of exertion of energy from exercise to socializing. While summer Dryness can be beneficial, such as drying out firewood that can then be used to keep us warm during winter or drying out an overly Stagnant or Relaxed condition, too much Dryness can make us feel worn down and completely depleted. We can bring moisture and shade to our inner landscapes through summer's cooling emollient remedies such as Rose (*Rosa* spp.) and Aloe Vera (*Aloe vera*). We can also pay attention to the ways fluid is being moved around and stored in our body by supporting the various rivers, lakes, deltas, and oceans of our inner landscape through cardiovascular tonics, diuretics, and water-rich plants and fruits. If you live in a place where summers are muggier, you can draw on the beneficial qualities of Dryness through astringent herbs and circulatory tonics such as Yarrow (*Achillea millefolium*) and Sage (*Salvia officinalis*).

As a season of youth, with all of its hormonal fluctuations and adventures in self-discovery, summer can be beneficial for learning about herbal approaches to hormonal health as well as working with herbs that support hormonal balance such as Red Clover (*Trifolium pratense*), Nettles (*Urtica dioica*), and Motherwort (*Leonurus cardiaca*). Summer is also a time of supporting our heart's blossoming and the cardiovascular system. It can be a powerful season to reconnect with your youthful energy and dreams, since as we get older there is a benefit to inner youth work in the same way inner child work benefits our healing practices.


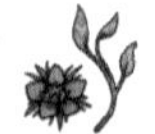

Within Western esoteric tradition, fire is a symbol of inspiration and creativity, sparking ideas and inspiration, and we can support the sparks of summer's bonfire by working with plant allies encouraging vision and imagination. While any plant ally of ours can enhance our creativity, there are some plants with a reputation for keeping the creative fires burning. Peppermint (*Mentha piperita*) wakes us up to our creative energy, while Sage (*Salvia officinalis*) and Rose (*Rosa* spp.) are guides to the multilayered quality of creative wisdom. The land in summer reflects the patterns of our own effort to make something with our dreams and plant allies, helping us straddle the waking and dreaming worlds and navigate our own bright becoming.

# *Summer Plant Allies*

## Calendula

*(Calendula officinalis)*

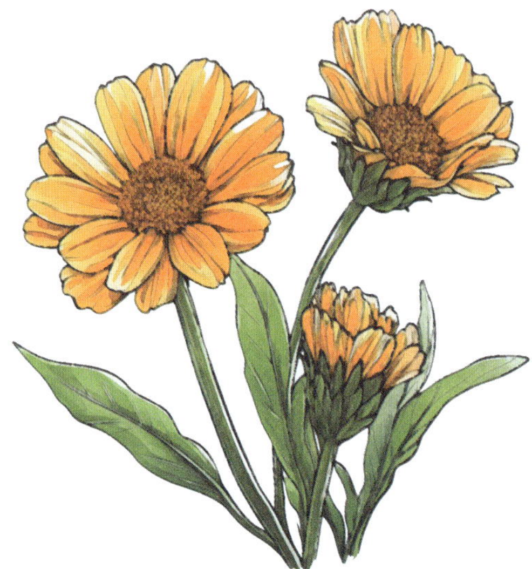

**Common + Folk Names:** Pot marigold, ruggles, holigold, gowan, bull's eye, Mary bud, ringelblume, summer's bride, spousa solis

**Elements:** Fire, earth

**Zodiac Signs:** Embodies the energy of Taurus, Leo, and Sagittarius. A remedy for Virgo and Sagittarius

**Planets:** Sun, Venus

**Moon Phase:** Full moon

**Part Used:** Flower

**Habitat:** Native to Eurasia but found worldwide

**Growing Conditions:** Full sun and thrives in a variety of soil types.

**Collection:** Collect the flowers as they bloom. Deadheading the plant will guarantee flowers for much of the growing season.

**Flavor:** Bitter, pungent

**Temperature:** Cool to warm

**Moisture:** Dry

**Tissue States:** Cold, Heat

**Actions:** Alterative, antibacterial, antifungal, anti-inflammatory, antispasmodic, antiviral, astringent, calmative, choleretic, demulcent, diaphoretic, emmenagogue, immunostimulant, probiotic, vulnerary

**Contraindications:** Generally regarded as safe, but avoid during pregnancy because of emmenagogue qualities. No drug interactions known, but use caution with sedatives, antihypertensives, and insulin medications.

**Dosage:** Standard dosage

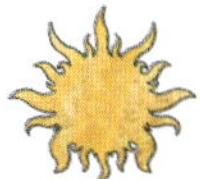

Calendula is one of the first flowers to bloom on the land I live with. A prized healer of wounds, batches of its sunny-colored salve can be used on all variety of skin-healing needs, from simple cuts to recovery from surgical procedures. Calendula promotes the formation of granulation tissues, and in addition to its repairing qualities, the herb protects against infections like *E. coli* and staph by stimulating the production of white blood cells.[7] Overall, it brings restorative sunlight to the body and spirit after a period of unwanted damp and darkness.

As an anti-inflammatory and febrifuge, Calendula reduces fever and can be included in herbal baths and teas for feverish children as well as adults. The flower is a great plant to have in your apothecary for all sorts of childhood needs, from colds and fevers, upset stomachs (including diarrhea), and skin issues from rashes to acne. It's also a good herb to include in post-illness restorative blends for all ages, especially if the illness was lingering or someone is recovering from a chronic condition.

Calendula excels at reducing signs of excess heat and inflammation when combined with damp stagnation. Some of the signs of damp heat are swollen glands, including lymph nodes; congestion, both digestive and in the upper respiratory system; a feeling of overfullness; and thirst without a strong impulse to drink. In addition to sluggish digestion, Calendula can help with heavy periods and cramping.

Topically, the herb is used for wound care, including as an oil, compress, liniment, herbal wash, and hydrosol. It is a well-loved and effective vulnerary, helping skin and tissue heal after damage from cuts and bruises to acne and sunburn. Use as a gargle for gingivitis and mouth sores, in nasal washes for sinus infections and nosebleeds, as well as in an eyewash for conjunctivitis and tired, irritated, or scratched eyes. It's useful as a compress for eyestrain from staring at screens too long.

Calendula is useful in treating varicose veins, leg ulcers and abscesses, and ringworm, as well as aiding the skin after exposure to the elements, including sun- and windburn and general air pollution. For animal and insect bites, it can be used topically and internally to prevent infections. Those who are suffering from sore nipples while nursing can find relief through Calendula compresses followed by application of the herbal oil. You can also include the herb in sitz baths for hemorrhoid relief and postpartum care and as a douche for vaginal infections.

### Seasonal Uses

As one of the first flowers to bloom in spring, I use Calendula as a circulatory tonic in daily teas to move energy throughout the body after the slowness of winter. In summer, a Calendula salve tucked into a small first-aid kit whenever we are out and about can bring relief to skin irritations, including insect bites, as well as help us recover from exposure to the elements. For autumn, Calendula staves off and shortens the length of colds, preventing and helping in the recovery from infections that can increase as the weather grows cooler and we move more indoors. Calendula is one of my favorite herbs to add to baths and shower rinses for the long nights of winter, acting as a little floral representation of the sun while keeping the skin healthy and glowing.

### Magickal Uses

Calendula appears on altars from India to Mexico as a beautiful plant offering. Scott Cunningham recommends picking the flowers in the middle of the day under bright sunlight to create charms to strengthen and gladden the heart.[8] Cunningham also describes a curious tradition whereby if a girl walks barefoot on Calendula she'll understand the language of birds—indicating the flower may be useful for folk with avian familiars.[9]

Garlands of these protective flowers can be hung throughout the home to keep out unwanted energies and spirits. Add the petals to dream bundles to aid you in your night visions and psychic dreaming. Greek tradition used Calendula as a symbol of "fond memories and good wishes."[10]

### The Calendula Personality

Calendula folk are those who have been told on many occasions that they are "a bit too much." Many of us will experience being told at least once that something about us is "too much"—often a form of microaggression pointing out our perceived "otherness" as a problem to be managed and hidden away. For Calendula folk, their experience of hearing they are "too much," and even being punished for this, has led them to adopt a protective energy that dulls their brightness and hides it away behind a veneer of brashness, feigned invulnerability, or an exhausting game of trying to keep hidden, which comes off as shyness to those around them. None of these expressions feel authentic to Calendula folk but are simply the masks they have developed to keep themselves safe. Working with Calendula can allow us to reconnect to authentic self-expression without shame for the greater intensity of feeling, experience, and expressiveness we might have in comparison with our peers. Calendula helps folks learn moderation when necessary but, more importantly, open back up to the warmth and shelter of close relationships. Calendula supports us in making wise decisions on who we relate to through accepting the beauty of our intensity and sensitivity, lighting the way for us to find others who resonate with our brightness.

# Milky Oat

*(Avena sativa)*

**Common + Folk Names:** Dousar, haver, goldes, ruddes, pot marigold

**Elements:** Water, earth

**Zodiac Signs:** Embodies the energy of Pisces.
A remedy for all signs.

**Planets:** Moon, Venus, Jupiter

**Moon Phase:** New moon

**Parts Used:** Unripe seeds (milky oats) and stem (oatstraw)

**Habitat:** An annual grass that has naturalized throughout much of North America and is indigenous to Europe, Asia, and northern Africa

**Growing Conditions:** Full sun and rich soil with moderate water

**Collection:** Collect the Milky Oat tops in early spring, when they excrete "milk" when squeezed.

**Flavor:** Sweet

**Temperature:** Neutral to Warm

**Moisture:** Moist

**Tissue States:** Tension, Cold, Dryness



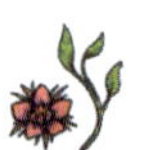

**Actions:** Antidepressant, alterative, demulcent, diaphoretic, nervine, nutritive, reproductive tonic, diuretic, endocrine tonic

**Contraindications:** Generally regarded as safe

**Dosage:** Standard dosage

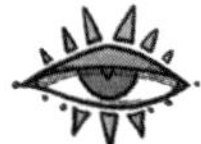

Milky Oat is one of the best examples of a long-term trophorestorative for the nervous system. The herb is a favored remedy for folks who feel like their energy and their focus are scattered far and wide. For sensitive folks and especially empaths, a sign that Milky Oat might be a good option is when they are feeling a million emotional sound bites at once from everyone around them. Milky Oat is also great for dealing with information overload (pair with *Scutellaria lateriflora*) and compassion fatigue when we're not only exhausted by what is happening in our immediate environment but from events around the world.

Milky Oat has a combination of qualities useful for folks in all stages of life suffering from nervous tension, whether brought on by anxiety, depression, injury, overwork, or trauma. The herb is a mild antidepressant and increases energy without being overstimulating, which is especially helpful when low moods are accompanied by insomnia. It is useful for those recovering from drug and alcohol addiction as it will rebalance their worn-out nervous systems. Seniors benefit from Milky Oat, especially if they are experiencing paralysis and chronic fatigue. The herb is great for convalescence and recovery after a period of debilitation whether from the flu, long-term illness, or a heightened period of stress and anxiety. Milky Oat also aids with digestion, especially constipation, as it is mucilaginous and can assist with the passage of stools.

In traditional western herbalism, Milky Oat has been in use for a long time, and 12th-century herbalist, writer, composer, and mystic Hildegard von Bingen wrote about it in her book *Physica* and its affect on mental health. Using the language of the time, Hildegard describes using Milky Oat this way:

*But let whoever is worn out with paralysis and as a result has a split mind and empty thoughts . . . be in a sweat bath when the wheat in the hot water in which it has been cooked is poured over the hot stones. Let them do this often; they will return to themselves and gain sanity.*[11]

Her description aligns with modern use: Milky Oat is rebalancing to the nervous system, helps in recovering energy after a period of debilitation, and acts as a general restorative tonic. Would a sweat bath as Hildegard described be useful today for supporting someone struggling with nervous exhaustion? Probably—sweat baths used to be much more common in traditional western herbalism and eclectic medicine, and the dynamic of sweating mixed with cold plunges has a lot of healing benefits. A hand, foot, or full-body bath of Milky Oat would be useful, too, if a sweat bath isn't an option.

Milky Oat's hormone-balancing qualities relieve tension headaches and melancholic states that might occur before and during menstruation as well as a variety of menopausal symptoms such as pain, exhaustion, and insomnia. The herb is great for postpartum, supporting all the big transitions of the fourth trimester.

High in silicon, Milky Oat is strengthening to hair, nails, teeth, and bones when used internally and externally. Milky Oat in baths or as part of an herbal oil blend relieves itchiness from skin conditions like eczema and psoriasis, lessens pain, and strengthens the skin's elasticity. Neuralgia, rheumatism, and fibromyalgia are all helped by Milky Oat.

### Seasonal Uses

In spring, I I carefully watch the Milky Oat patches, waiting for that brief moment when they are ripe and milky so that I can make a nourishing nervous system tincture to use all year as well as help with any post-winter convalescence. In summer, I add Milky Oat to cool teas to feel balanced and easy in the heat. The busyness of autumn can pull us in all sorts of directions, but a daily tonic of Milky Oat keeps us focused on our intentions, connected to our intuition, and feeling nourished through our wisdom. I love combining Milky Oat with oatmeal baths to nourish dry skin in the winter and lift spirits during the long dark of the season.



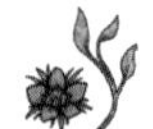

### Magickal Uses

While there is not a lot of magickal folklore regarding Milky Oat, the nutritive and abundant qualities of the herb hint of its magickal uses, which are primarily for prosperity and abundance rituals. I find the plant to have a special affinity for lunar energy and especially the energy of the new moon, helping us deal with life's ever-changing experiences.

### The Milky Oat Personality

The Milky Oat person is exhausted—completely and utterly. They feel debilitated, unable to sleep but struggling to wake, and life can seem like a hazy, directionless dream. Unable to focus for long on any one thing, Milky Oat folks struggle to determine their sense of purpose in life. Their energy seems to be flung far and wide, but they struggle to recognize where to focus it and what to grow and harvest in their life. Even though they are exhausted, they can be excessive in the way they expend energy, finding themselves prone to chronic cycles of burnout. Part of the struggle of Milky Oat folks is that they are interested in and good at many things, yet fall prey to the idea of having to have a sudden epiphany of their singular purpose and calling, when life is a series of experiments and realizations, full of many paths and callings. Some Milky Oat folks even seek out or overuse psychedelic drugs in an attempt to access an "instant breakthrough." The beauty of Milky Oat folks, though, is that they are good at so many things, and this is a profound gift! They have an abundance of energy when it is held gently and with focused intent. Working with Milky Oat helps them to weave the diversity of their passions into an interconnected melody of calling.

# Nettles

*(Urtica dioica)*

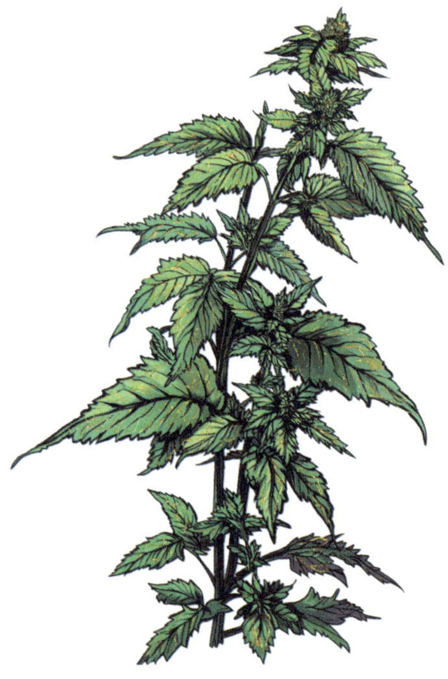

**Common + Folk Names:** Stinging nettle, wild spinach, beesting nettle, devil's leaf, hidgy-pidgy, hoky-poky

**Element:** Fire

**Zodiac Signs:** Embodies the energy of Aries and Scorpio. A remedy for Scorpio, Capricorn, and Pisces.

**Planet:** Mars

**Moon Phase:** Waxing quarter moon

**Parts Used:** Leaves, seeds, roots, and young tops

**Habitat:** Just about everywhere

**Growing Conditions:** Grow in wet, rich soil—think compost heaps and old manure.

**Collection:** Cut three to four inches off the early spring plants. Seeds can be collected in the early fall when plants are brown.

**Flavor:** Salty, slightly bitter

**Temperature:** Cool

**Moisture:** Dry

**Tissue States:** Cold, Stagnation, Dryness

**Actions:** Alterative, antihistamine, antirheumatic, anti-inflammatory, astringent, blood tonic, circulation stimulant, decongestant, diuretic,

expectorant, hemostatic, hypoglycemic, hypotensive, immunostimulant, nutritive, vasodilator, thyroid tonic, antiseptic

**Contraindications:** Nettle leaf is generally considered safe. Do not take root during pregnancy. Use with caution with blood thinners.

**Dosage:** Standard dosage

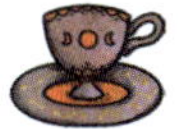

Nettles are a beloved panacea, good for just about everything. As a wonderfully nutritive herb, Nettles nourish the entire body with a broad range of vitamins and minerals that support energetic flow, awareness, and resiliency.

Nettles are a strengthening herb to use when a person's constitution is weak or weakened, such as in cases of anemia, a weak digestive system, and especially during convalescence. The herb helps increase energy and overcome fatigue as well as restore a worn-down emotional system. Nettles strengthen the kidneys and adrenal glands, activate the metabolism, nourish the liver and blood, and improve elasticity of veins. The diuretic and anti-inflammatory actions of Nettles are also useful in treating rheumatism and gout. The herb enlivens the immune system, and in spring you can even cook the young greens like spinach. Nettles are one of my favorite antihistamines and anti-inflammatories and can be useful in cases of seasonal allergies, asthma, acne, eczema, and food allergies.

Nettles have an affinity for the blood, improving circulation and offering a rich source of iron. They are also useful in reducing blood sugar levels and balancing blood pressure. For menstruation, Nettles alleviate heavy and prolonged periods. You can also use Nettles to stop nosebleeds and excess bleeding both internally and externally. Nettles have a strong relationship with the kidneys, stimulating sluggish kidneys, alleviating edema, and generally cleansing the fluids of the body.

During pregnancy, Nettles, in combination with other herbs such as Raspberry Leaf (*Rubus idaeus*), are a wonderful daily multivitamin for a parent and growing fetus. Use in postpartum especially if there was postpartum hemorrhage. Nettles support nursing parents by increasing milk if there is too little or reducing milk production if there is too much.

For the reproductive systems, Nettle root has been used to treat prostatitis, vaginitis, and vaginal discharges. If infertility is an issue, Nettles are useful for nourishing and revitalizing the body attempting to conceive. If low libido, erectile dysfunction, or general sexual anxiety is present, Nettles resettle and center the nervous system (combine with *Avena sativa*). Use during menopause for night sweats by taking as a tea before bed combined with Sage (*Salvia officinalis*). The root also reduces prostate enlargement.

As an antihistamine, Nettles strengthen the outer membranes of cells, which makes them less vulnerable to inflammation and allergic reactions.[12] Nettles can also be used in cases of eczema, hay fever, asthma, acne, and food allergies.

Use externally as an oil or wash for bedsores, diaper rash, burns and wounds, and brittle nails, and to treat the sting of Nettles. Traditional use includes hitting arthritic joints with fresh Nettles to alleviate pain and stiffness. I have found Nettles to be good (both internally and externally) for growing pains of all sorts, both emotional and physical.

### Seasonal Uses

Nettles are a great spring medicine—they warm up the digestive fires and rebuild energy after winter as well as build up our histamine resistance. In the summer, I turn to Nettles as a source of electrolytes, helping keep me steady and hydrated during long stretches of heat. In autumn, it's once again useful to keep Nettles in daily rotation for seasonal allergies as well as a gentle immunostimulant to protect against colds. Nettles warm the body and promote circulation, strengthening the blood and protecting against stagnation throughout the winter months.

### Magickal Uses

Nettles are very protective and can return harmful energy to the sender. Use as a protective powder around the boundaries of the house. Nettles enhance the energy of fire and all forms of candle magick. Toss in the Midsummer bonfire before jumping over the flames to burn away unwanted energy and surround


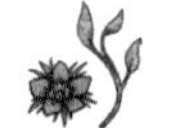

yourself with protection. The herb also has a traditional use in blends for courage.[13]

### The Nettles Personality

The Nettles personality struggles to live in the moment. They are often dazed, brain-fogged, and worn down. Many are simply going through the motions of their day; the little pleasant details of life are simply a blur, passing by unappreciated. There can be a lingering feeling of sadness, wariness, and uncertainty. The blur and sameness of it all can make a Nettles person feel they are boundaryless but not in an expansive and blissful sort of way. They can get walked all over by others and begin to feel resentful for not being appreciated.

Fortunately, Nettles help bring us rapidly back to the moment. (Think about how their sting does just that when you accidentally stumble upon them.) For the muddled and unmoored, a healthy recentering can go a long way in feeling better. In addition, Nettles help us set boundaries with ourselves, which, in turn, allows us to set healthy boundaries with others. With the heat and stimulation of Nettles, the fog can lift and the excitement of life come rushing back in, allowing Nettles folk to bring their expansiveness to any project or relationship they involve themselves in.

# The Summer Apothecary

## Cooling Off: Supporting the Body After Sun Exposure

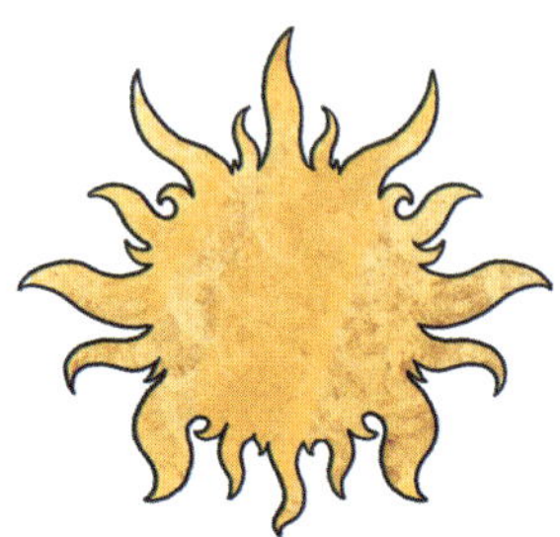

### *Herbal Actions*

*Cooling, anti-inflammatory, alterative, emollient, and demulcent*

At the risk of sounding like an after-school commercial, the best way to stay sun-safe is to stay sun-smart. Stick to the shade during the hottest parts of the day, keep hydrated, wear sunscreen and/or cool protective layers, and respect the power of the sun. The following plants are great friends for cooling off (and not burning out) after long summer days.

**Aloe Vera (*Aloe barbadensis/Aloe vera*):** One of the most frequently used herbs of my childhood, Aloe Vera is a trusted topical plant ally to use after a day spent in the sun. The inner gel is cooling and moistening, alleviating inflammation in the body both internally and externally. Along with sunburn, indications for Aloe Vera include feeling overheated after sun exposure even without a sunburn, as well as general burns, rashes, allergic skin reactions, and eczema.

**Borage (*Borago officinalis*)**: These beautiful blue flowers and their prickly leaves help to balance heat and cold in the body. Indications include feelings of "summer

sadness" from overextending yourself emotionally and physically, dehydration (add flowers to water), brain fog, and general anxiety.

**Lavender (*Lavandula* spp.):** A great cooling plant ally to keep on hand, especially as a body rinse, spray, or compress after heat exposure. Indications include nausea, irritability, tension headaches, and all varieties of skin complaints such as heat rash, insect bites and stings, burns, wounds, and so on.

**Lemon Balm (*Melissa officinalis*):** If you've overdone it in the heat and find yourself dealing with heat exhaustion, Lemon Balm can be a great ally to have at hand. In addition to drinking *room-temperature* tea to recover from heat exhaustion, I like to use it as part of a cool compress at the wrists and back of the neck. If I know I'll be out in the heat or likely to get bugbites, I make a jar of Lemon Balm tea at the beginning of the day so that when I get back home it'll be ready for me to drink or use in compresses. Indications include social burnout, tension headaches, and heart palpitations.

**Milky Oat (*Avena sativa*):** For those who experience a spike in stress after sun exposure or who've overexerted themselves, Milky Oat helps to nourish the body, especially the nervous system. Indications include muscle weakness and soreness, low energy, itchy skin conditions, and nervous palpitations.

**Peppermint (*Mentha piperita*):** Peppermint cools the body, softens stress, and improves focus, all helpful qualities when recovering from the heat. Indications include signs of trapped heat, brain fog and lack of focus, summer colds, indigestion, and heartburn.

**Rose (*Rosa* spp.):** Beautiful Rose is a prized cooling summer skin ally. It can be used as a skin wash post-sun as well as in your daily skincare routine. Rose hydrosol is one of my favorite year-round skin treatments, especially in the summer. Indications for Rose include sunburn, heat rash, dizziness, anxiety, and general inflammation.

# Unbothered: Caring for the Skin during the Summer Months against Bugs, Bumps & More

## *Herbal Actions*

*Anti-inflammatory, alterative, liver tonics, and nervines*

Some of the first herbal remedies I made were topical herbal oils for use on the bruises and sore muscles I sustained as a student athlete. While I was impressed by the results, it was the process of creating these special blends, applying them, and taking care of myself in ways I didn't always feel looked out for as an athlete that I really loved. For me, working with plant allies to care for our body's largest organ, the skin, has remained an act of profound self-care.

**Catnip (*Nepeta cataria*):** A very-effective mosquito repellent, Catnip can be used throughout the day on the skin to keep away biting bugs. Indications include existing in a world with mosquitoes.

**Lavender (*Lavandula* spp.):** Lavender is one of the few essential oils I use on a regular basis because it is so helpful for reducing the itch and discomfort of bugbites. The essential oil can be applied directly to the skin (for most essential oils this is not safe). I also use compresses of the flowers to heal skin from bumps, bruises, bites, and rashes, as well as adding it to herbal baths and using it as a hydrosol. Indications for Lavender include general skin complaints, especially with muscle pain.

**Milky Oat (*Avena sativa*):** If you're struggling with the increased sensation that bugbites and stings can bring, using Milky Oat internally (tea or tincture) can calm the nervous system and regulate your sensory feedback.

**Mullein (*Verbascum thapsus*):** The giant leaves of Mullein are great for those with dry skin. Indications include signs of dryness and heat (including joint pain and sciatica) and inflamed skin conditions like eczema, boils, burns, and ulcers.

**Plantain (*Plantago major, P. lanceolata*):** With a beesting, the first plant I look for is Plantain, and if I'm lucky, I'll find a leaf, crush it up, and apply it to the site of pain and swelling. Plantain heals damaged tissue, alleviates pain, and assists with


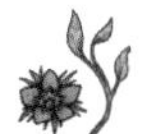

wound care. Indications include all varieties of stings and bites, especially when there is hard and painful swelling.

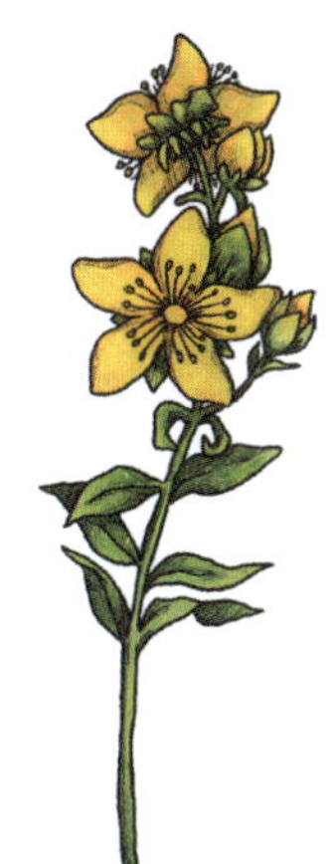

**St. Joan's Wort (*Hypericum perforatum*):** I like using a combination of St. Joan's Wort and Rose (*Rosa* spp.) herbal oil as a post-sun skin treatment as well as for bumps and bruises. You can add a few drops of Lavender essential oil if you're also dealing with mosquito bites. I like to apply the herbal oil after a shower to preserve the natural oils on my skin or after spraying my skin with a floral hydrosol. Indications for St. Joan's Wort include sun exposure and a burned-out nervous system with stress aggravated by bites.

## Opening Up: Nourishing the Heart

### *Herbal Actions*

*Cardiotonics, circulatory tonics, and nervines*

Any season can be a time of opening up the heart, but there is something about the expectation of adventuring, dreaming, and socializing in summer that calls for extra herbal support for issues of the heart. While the following plant allies work to heal the physical heart, I primarily focus on herbs for the emotional experiences of the heart—which will, in turn, support the actual organ.

**Hawthorn (*Crataegus monogyna*):** Hawthorn is one of the most prized cardiotonics in traditional western herbalism, and I've used it for a wide range of heart health needs, including reducing the stress that caused heart issues in the first place. Hawthorn helps us to love again after heartbreak, guiding us to trust our heart again. Indications include minor palpitations and rhythm irregularities caused by stress, fear of emotional vulnerability, and someone trying to hide away their brightness.

**Motherwort (*Leonurus cardiaca*):** I was introduced to Motherwort as a "hug in a bottle," speaking to the plant's ability to make us feel comforted as if by the most

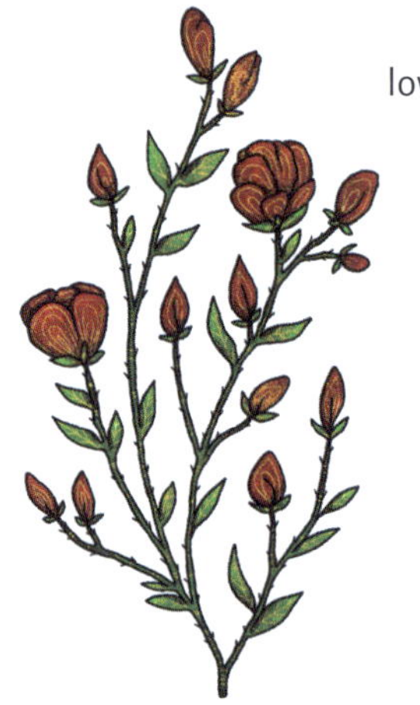

loving of parents, real or imagined. Indications for Motherwort include heightened impatience and irritability, folks who had to grow up too fast, and tired-out caregivers.

**Rose (*Rosa* spp.):** Rose is my favorite heart-opening, love-supporting herb because it protects us while softening the hard edges of our emotional experiences in all the right ways. Indications include general restlessness, struggles with shame, unresolved anger, and memory issues tied to heartbreak.

## Shining Clearly: Managing Seasonal Allergies

For an overview of seasonal allergy support, please refer to the Balance section in the Spring Apothecary, but following are a few of my favorite summertime herbs for allergy relief.

**Butterbur (*Petasites hybridus*):** A lovely antihistamine, Butterbur works best when you start to take it a few weeks before allergy season arrives. Indications include asthma, hay fever, allergy-induced headaches, and skin conditions brought on or aggravated by allergies.

**Goldenrod (*Solidago* spp.):** Goldenrod is a great choice of antihistamine when allergies manifest as sinusitis, respiratory inflammation, and excess mucus. Further indications include asthma, stagnant digestion, and adrenal fatigue.

**Yarrow (*Achillea millefolium*):** While you can use Yarrow as a tea, tincture, or capsule, the flowers and leaves are one of my favorite topical treatments as a steam for allergy relief, alleviating allergy-related headaches, asthma, and congestion. Indications include water retention, poor circulation, low energy, red splotchiness of the skin, conditions that worsen in air-conditioned environments, and exposure to environmental pollutants (including wildfire smoke).

## The Fertile Land: Supporting Reproductive Fertility & Conception

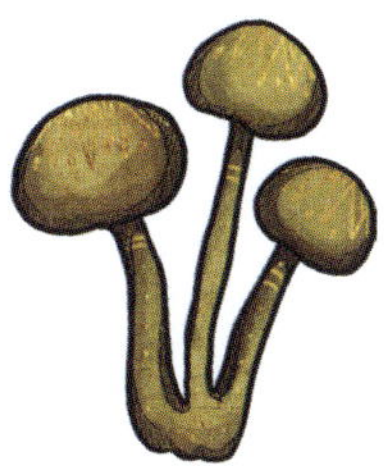

Summer represents a time of growth and fertility throughout the land, and if you are seeking to support your own fertility, there are a number of plant allies to call upon. Fertility can be complex, so if you're having difficulty conceiving, you should work with an herbalist specializing in reproductive health. The following are general reproduction tonics and helpful for most folks, but you should also invite at least one nervine into your herbal protocol to alleviate stress.

**Ashwagandha (*Withania somnifera*):** A great nervine for all partners involved in the fertility process, Ashwagandha supports both internal and external reproductive organs and general hormonal health and alleviates stress. Indications include fatigue, low sperm count, and low libido.

**Damiana (*Turnera diffusa*):** This plant carries both the best qualities of herbal aphrodisiacs and the nourishing and restorative qualities of an adaptogen. One reason Damiana is so effective as an aphrodisiac is that it reduces stress and stress-related complaints, and as an adaptogen the herb works to regulate the pituitary gland and increase energy. Indications include general fertility challenges, low libido, depression, low sperm count, and a desire to reconnect to sex as a pleasurable, low-stakes experience.

**Lady's Mantle (*Alchemilla vulgaris*):** A great uterine tonic, Lady's Mantle preps the uterus for conception, balances menstrual cycles, and supports healthy ovulation and fertility. Indications include weak pelvic floor muscles, fibroids, pelvic inflammation, and excess heat and tension.

**Rose (*Rosa* spp.):** Rose is a beautiful aphrodisiac that helps us relax into sensual experiences on our own terms, protected and open. The herb also supports some of the practical considerations of fertility, increasing sperm count and regulating menses. Indications include low energy, stress around intimacy, irregular menses, and low sperm count.

**Saw Palmetto (*Serenoa repens*):** An excellent adaptogen and general hormonal tonic, Saw Palmetto helps with both internal and external reproductive organs from uterine and testicular atrophy to general pelvic congestion. The herb is especially supportive in cases of low sperm count, erectile dysfunction, and prostatitis. Indications include low sexual energy, chronic immune weakness, and general appearance of weakness.

## Happy Belly: Herbs for Stomach Health

In traditional western herbalism, the stomach is the seat of our internal fire, and tending to this inner heat is one of the cornerstones of our practice. The following herbs help with some of the most common digestive complaints, not only of the stomach but the whole digestive system, so that you can have a happy belly all year long.

**Chamomile (*Matricaria chamomilla*):** My favorite stomach tonic for children young and old, Chamomile is a gentle but effective remedy for many varieties of indigestion. Indications include colic, indigestion caused by emotional upset, grumpiness, brain fog, and diarrhea.

**Fennel (*Foeniculum vulgare*):** For those who run hot but still need help with their digestive fire without overheating, Fennel is a great plant ally. Keeping a packet of Fennel seeds with you on your summer travels to chew on after meals is a great indigestion preventative. Indications include bloating, burping and gas, and general tension after eating.

 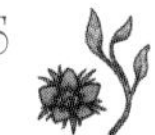 

**Licorice (*Glycyrrhiza glabra*):** A general gut tonic and restorative to the digestive system, Licorice is an excellent ally for those struggling with digestive problems due to endocrine system issues. Indications include inflammation of the digestive system, including gastritis, hiccups, stomach acidity, and motion sickness.

**Marshmallow (*Althea officinalis*):** This is a balancing herb that synergizes all body systems. Excellent for all forms of stomach and digestive issues arising from inflammation, including colitis and diarrhea. Indications include gastritis, irritable bowel syndrome (IBS), dysbiosis, heartburn, hemorrhoids, and general inflammation.

**Turmeric (*Curcuma longa*):** My favorite digestive tonic is *haldi doodh*, or golden milk, for making us feel warm, nourished, grounded, and centered. Turmeric helps us digest and absorb nutrients and lower blood sugar and can be enjoyed as part of a pre-meal bitters blend. The golden root also aids in expelling worms and parasites as well as protecting and promoting growth of healthy gut flora. Indications include abdominal pain and bloating, IBS, indigestion, poor digestion and absorption of nutrients, dull skin, and issues stemming from inflammation.

## Adventures Far & Wide: Plant Allies for Travel

Keeping a small kit of plant remedies with you when traveling allows you to address many issues you may encounter. While your kit will be dependent on the unique needs of you and your travel group, as well as where you're going, the following are some of my favorite travel companions for most adventures.

**Ginger (*Zingiber officinale*):** One of my favorite herbs to prevent motion sickness, Ginger is helpful for general indigestion, protecting against infections, and adjusting to new time zones and environments. Indications include low energy, poor circulation (including caused by travel conditions), and loss of or low appetite.

**Lemon Balm (*Melissa officinalis*):** An overall great tonic herb to have around, Lemon Balm is antimicrobial, antiviral, antihistamine, and a lovely digestive tonic, all qualities you want in a plant ally travel companion. Indications include general fatigue, social exhaustion, mental weariness, and restlessness.

**Licorice (*Glycyrrhiza glabra*):** I carry a few teabags of Licorice root with me in my travel kit to support digestive health and help with food poisoning, as an immunomodulator, and as an overall rejuvenative tonic. Licorice is also a great remedy for motion sickness. Indications include digestive upset, low energy, allergies, headache, and general jet lag.

**Plantain (*Plantago major, P. lanceolata*):** I keep a small tin of Plantain salve in my travel kit not only for beestings and bugbites, but for bumps, bruises, and general wound care. See the Unbothered section for indications.

**Skullcap (*Scutellaria lateriflora*):** Travel asks for a lot of focus when getting from one place to another, and Skullcap is one of my favorite herbs for quieting anxiety and promoting clearheadedness. It is also a great ally to induce sleep and to help us feel better if we happen to catch a cold. Indications include mental fatigue, loss of focus, physical exhaustion, tension headaches, and indigestion.

## Vigor & Strength: Building Up the Blood

The idea of "building up the blood" is an old one in traditional western herbalism and has been used to describe remedies for conditions like anemia, but also broader neurological diseases and early concepts of mental health conditions. Blood is considered the seat of vitality and health, so weakened blood, producing a condition like anemia where there is a low blood cell count and lack of oxygenation, would lead to poor health. This "weak blood" would be treated by building up the blood through iron-rich herbs, but also lifestyle changes such as improving the diet, getting good movement, accessing fresh air and green spaces, and engaging with emotionally and mentally fulfilling activities. As summer is traditionally


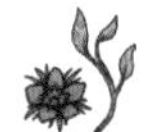

seen as a time of fire and the weather lends itself to a beneficial "blood-building" atmosphere, I want to highlight iron- and nutrient-rich herbs that can make us feel invigorated, strong, and full of vitality.

**Burdock (*Arctium lappa*):** A great herb to use when "congested blood" has led to skin imbalances such as boils, acne, eczema, and rashes. One of the primary indications for Burdock is excess heat and conditions that worsen in the heat, as the root helps to clear out congested heat from the liver, kidneys, and blood. Other indications include a low appetite, gas, and a general feeling of malaise.

**Dandelion (*Taraxacum officinale*):** If you're dealing with issues of elimination, slow digestion, and a sluggish liver and kidneys, Dandelion is a great plant to work with. It dissolves excess uric acid in the blood and urine, preventing painful buildup, as well as supporting the production of bile in the gallbladder and liver to aid digestion. An iron-rich ally, indications for Dandelion include chronic inflammation, stiff neck, excessive sweat, poor digestion, and symptoms that get better when moving or receiving bodywork.

**Nettles (*Urtica dioica*):** Nettles are the classic iron-rich, blood-building herb. They are gentle enough to be taken over a long period of time and often referred to as "nature's multivitamin" because of the plant's high vitamin and mineral content. The fresh or dried herb is best, but if you want to create an extract, use vinegar as your menstruum instead of alcohol to better draw out Nettles' minerals. Indications for Nettles include your classic signs of anemia: general fatigue, low color in the skin, lightheadedness, brittle hair and nails, and heart palpitations. Additional indications include water retention, acne, eczema, and general adrenal stress.

## The Youth of the Year: Herbs for Teens & Young Adults

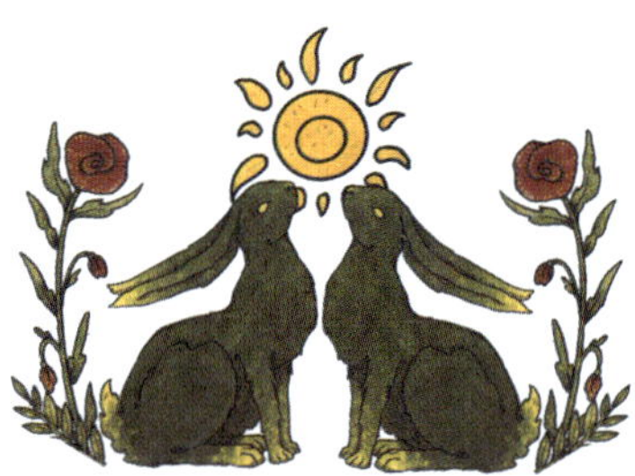

As a season traditionally associated with teens and young adults, summer flourishes in a dance between childhood energy and expanding maturity. The following herbs are not only abundant in summer, but address many of the challenges and experiences of young people and their rapidly changing bodies. Be sure to also check out The Lunar Body (see page 162) for additional suggestions for menstrual support as well as Calling Life Back to the Land (page 226) for supporting normal fluctuations in mood. The following can also be used either in plant form or as flower essence for healing your inner youth.

**Holy Basil (*Ocimum tenuiflorum*):** A great overall tonic for the young, Holy Basil or Tulsi is an adaptogen that works to manage stress and stressful environments (hello, middle school and high school!), as well as alleviate common health conditions like acne, indigestion, and anxiety. Indications include anxiety, mild depression, low energy, gas and distention, low immunity, and acne made worse by stress.

**Linden (*Tilia x europaea*):** Linden is a gentle ally to the young, helping them find their community (combine with *Melissa officinalis*) and feel like they fit into the world. Indications include general nervousness, irritability and impatience, insomnia, headaches, and redness of the skin.

**Motherwort (*Leonurus cardiaca*):** A wonderful plant ally for young folk seeking to feel held and supported as they explore all of who they are, Motherwort is especially good for young people who hide their sensitivity behind a wall of anger and toughness. Indications include PMS that brings on feelings of agitation,



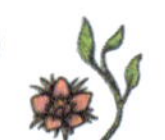

frustration, anger, and menstrual headaches; a sense of abandonment; and general anxiety around the complexity of growing up.

**Red Clover (*Trifolium pratense*):** One of my favorites to balance youthful hormones, Red Clover not only helps with skin issues like acne (use internally as a tea and externally as a wash), but has a gentle nourishing energy to settle emotions. Indications include acne, eczema, asthma, growing pains, and cold hands and feet.

**Skullcap (*Scutellaria lateriflora*):** Skullcap is a great plant ally for young people who need help quieting their heart and mind, focusing on tasks, and keeping everything in perspective. Indications include trouble falling asleep due to racing thoughts or anxiety, exam nerves, mood swings, and general stress.

**The Community Clinic in Summer**

*Cooling hydrosols to help with summer heat*

*Post-sun salves and liniments to soothe sunburn and heat rash*

*Bug sprays and salves to protect against and treat insect bites*

*Drawing powders and salves for thorns and stingers*

*Travel remedies like digestive aids, antinausea herbs, and general antiviral and antibacterial blends*

*Allergy remedies specific to summer complaints such as grass pollen and tree pollen*

*Circulatory tonics and cardiotonics to keep energy moving throughout the body to prevent conditions of excess heat*

# Summer Recipes & Rituals

## Energizing Summer Tea

Herbs like adaptogens, blood-building tonics, and uplifting nervines help us connect with summer's warmth without becoming burned out.

2 parts Holy Basil (*Ocimum tenuiflorum*)
1 part Nettles (*Urtica dioica*)
½ part Rosemary (*Salvia rosmarinus*)

## Soothing Summer Tea

For a soothing summer blend I recommend cooling nervines and adaptogens, anti-inflammatory herbs, and heart tonics. The following tea is based on one I first had when I briefly lived in Austin, Texas, but versions can be found throughout North Africa where Hibiscus (*Hibiscus* spp.) is a popular tea plant. It is especially good iced and sweetened.

3 parts Hibiscus (*Hibiscus* spp.)
½ part Peppermint (*Mentha piperita*)
Pinch of Cinnamon (*Cinnamomum* spp.)

## Nourishing Summer Tea

This nourishing blend incorporates heart-opening nervines and gentle digestive herbs that work with the energy of summer to help our inner landscape flourish during the longest days of the year.

2 part Nettles (*Urtica dioica*)
½ part Calendula (*Calendula officinalis*)
½ part Rose (*Rosa* spp.)

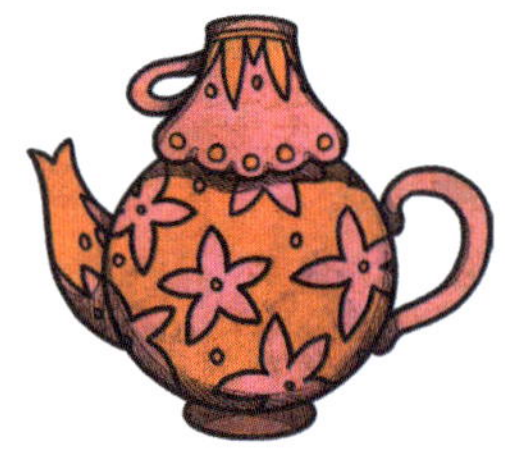

## Shelter Ritual

Sometimes we need to strengthen the boundaries of our spaces and call in protective and sheltering energy. The following ritual works with the energy of Mullein, a plant ally long associated with the power of Midsummer, witches, and protective magick, but you can substitute any protective plant. The spoken charm is a variety of old folk magick where things are spoken in one order and then reversed, creating a container of protection in all directions. Another dynamic of this ritual is calling in an energy of protection both around you and from within so that we can feel sheltered in both our inner and outer landscapes. If performing this ritual with a group, you can create an energizing call and response by having one part of the group say the first, fourth, seventh, and tenth lines and the other half of the group say the rest.

**You will need:**

Five candles—one for each direction and one for the center
Dried and ground Mullein (*Verbascum thapsus*)
Oil of choice for dressing the candles

Create your sacred space in your preferred way and begin by dressing the candles with the oil and dried Mullein, setting aside a small amount of Mullein to use later. Rub oil on the candles and then roll them in the Mullein, speaking to the spirit of Mullein your intention to call in protective and sheltering energy. Additionally, you can carve protective words or sigils on each candle, corresponding to each direction.

When the candles are prepared, place one in each cardinal direction and one in the center or on your altar with the set-aside Mullein.

Beginning in the east, light your candle and say

*East without* [hold your hands toward the east]
*East within* [hold your hands on your heart]
*I am sheltered and secure* [let your arms hang comfortably at your sides]

Continue with all of the directions in the same way.



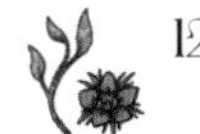

Light the center candle and say:

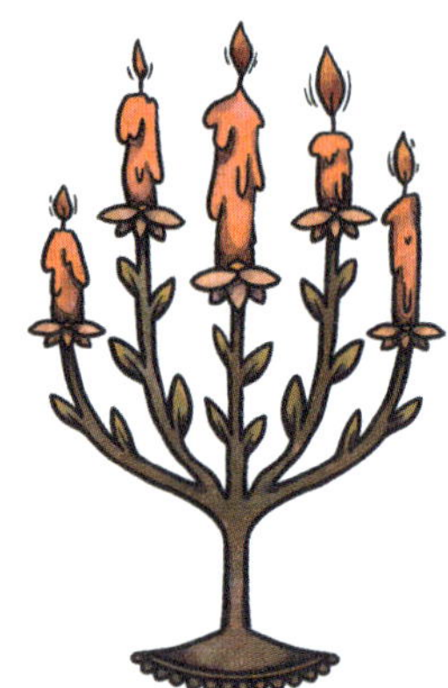

*North, East, South, West*
*Whenever I wake*
*Whenever I rest*
*By land, by sky, by fire, by sea*
*May I be sheltered*
*Wherever I be*
*By sea, by fire, by sky, by land*
*Protective powers*
*Ever at hand*
*West, South, East, North*
*I am protected*
*as I go forth!*

If it is safe to do so, let the candles continue to burn as you add the Mullein to a charm bag; the corners, windows, and doorways of your home; and/or to any personal mode of transportation such as shoes, mobility aids, bikes, or cars. Once done, extinguish the candles, and if you still have some Mullein left over, you can offer it as incense or return it to the earth.

## A Gratitude Blessing

A gratitude blessing helps us center in the abundance of the present moment and can be used as a personal blessing, a community prayer, or part of a larger ritual. Adapt the following blessing to either be singular or plural and change the seasonal reference to match your time of year:

*I am clear in this moment*
*that the fire of love runs through my veins*
*that when I struggle to see it*
*it burns brighter*
*pulling me home*
*to the warmth of shelter*
*of nourishment*
*of company*



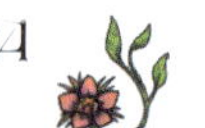

*of dreams*
*of hope*
*of creativity*
*of things I can't always name*
*but I know in this moment*
*bright as the summer sun*
*that the fire of love runs through my veins*
*steady and flowing*
*glowing and knowing*
*carrying me home again and again*
*blessed be*

## The Lover's Oracle

Choose three plant allies, whether the actual herb or a symbol:

one to represent your heart-body
one to represent your desire
one to represent your seeking self

Prepare your space, making a summer-inspired tea if you like, and lay your oracle of belonging out before you. Ground, center, and speak any divining charms you'd like. When ready, take up your herbs or objects, close your eyes, and either toss or place them at random on the oracle map. For summer, I like to toss herbs or charms up into the air above the oracle, connecting to the energetic nature of the season and letting them fall where they will.

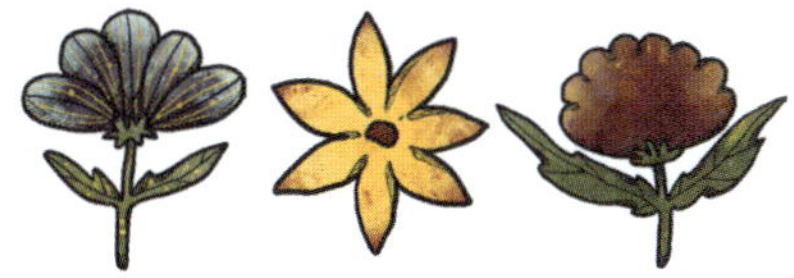

Where the heart herb or object lands speaks to the needs of your heart-body and the nourishing relationships between all parts of the land within and around you. The placement of your desire herb or object illuminates what it is you are desiring most in your life, as guided by your heart. The seeking self's placement represents the type of relationships of any variety you are looking for and choosing at this moment in your life.

Let's say your heart herb lands on the river of your oracle, representing movement in your life and the needs of your nervous system, suggesting perhaps your heart is feeling restless, led by a nervous system that's not quite settled. Your desire object may land in the mountain area, representing longevity, groundedness, and stability, pointing toward wanting more of this earthy energy in your life. Finally, the seeking self may land on the part of your oracle representing fire, heat, and action. There is a tension between these three parts of yourself—a heart that is restless, a desire for grounded stability, but a part of you still seeking quickness and heat.

From this oracle you might choose to pay closer attention to the types of relationships feeling nourishing but exciting to you, while working with plant allies to ground and center, so that your seeking feels less hurried and intense. Consider an herb that represents the need of your heart and nervous system to feel settled, one that is nutritive and grounding, and another that helps your seeking self to still feel invigorated and inspired but more at home in your body.

## The Waxing Quarter Moon

Within the astrological roots of traditional western herbalism, the waxing quarter moon is a time of hot and dry herbs, corresponding to the heat and dryness that come with long summer days. Summer embodies the energy of longevity, the shelter of community, and a land rich in abundance—each month throughout the year we can work with the waxing quarter moon to connect with the season of extended light.

In my own lunar practice, I enjoy timing my harvesting of plants and making remedies that correspond to the energies of strengthening, energizing, and awakening, including energy tonics, heart-strengthening blends, and circulatory tonics, with the waxing quarter moon.



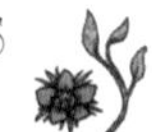

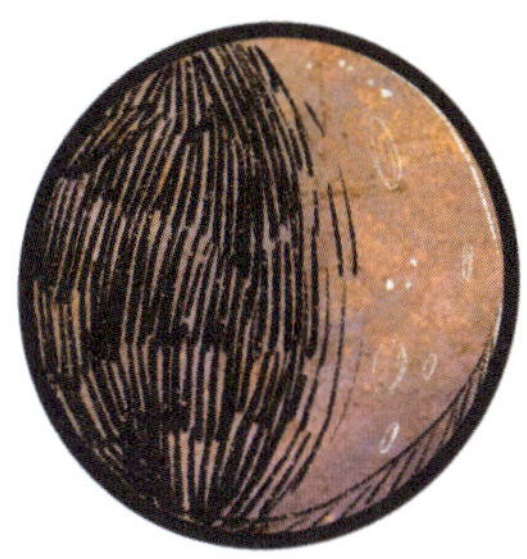

## *Waxing Quarter Moon Remedy Blessing*

To be said over remedies while making them, during their brewing process, or before administering them:

*By the light of the quarter moon*
*wax and grow*
*stir up energy*
*so healing may flow*

*as the moon sweeps wide*
*the remedy wakes*
*the glow of possibility*
*infuses in place*

*blessed be*

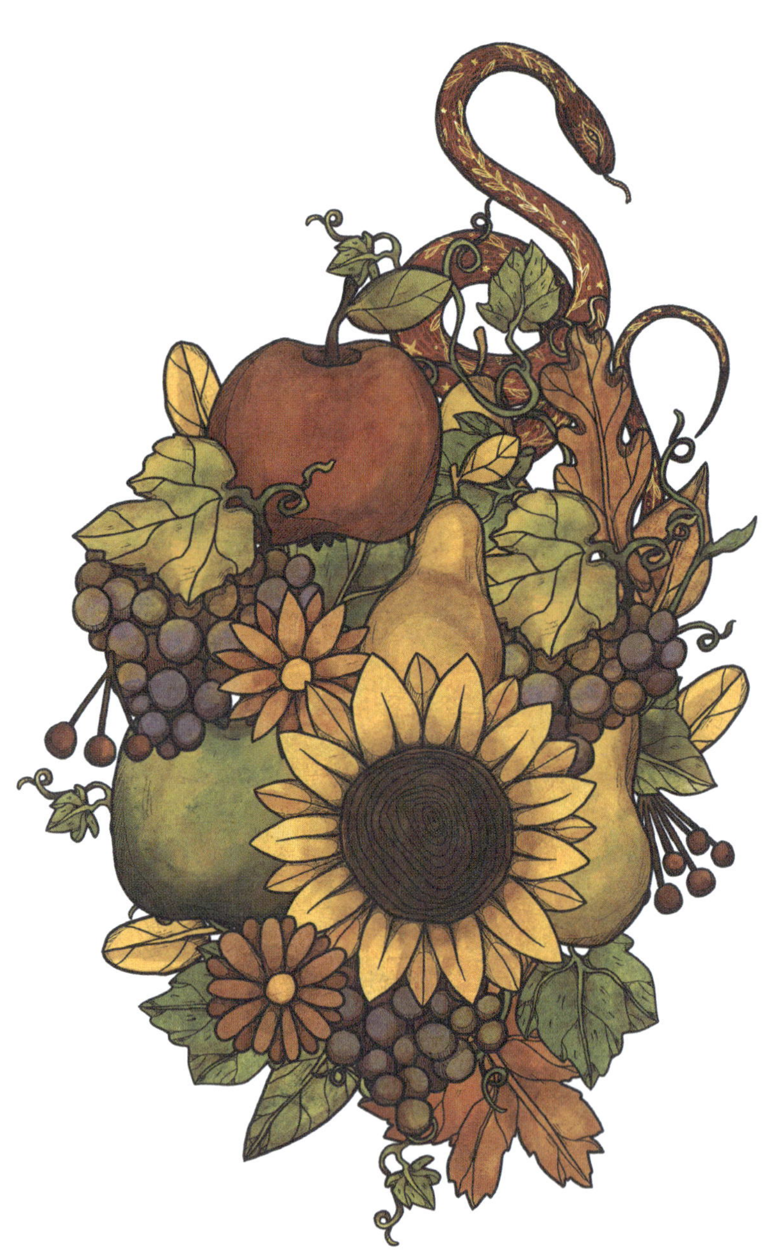

# Autumn

Summer sighs and autumn takes a deep breath in, pulling us from sun-dappled days to cooler mornings and even cooler nights. Autumn is a time of taking stock, tending to our boundary lands, and gathering at the end of harvest season to share in the abundance of community effort. The long slow yawn of summer's waning leaves the land in a liminal state, dancing between the bright and dark half of the year. With the ebbing of energy, autumn is a thinning time, where certain places in the landscape—between stone and branch, hollow and city block—become little doorways between the worlds.

Like bundled up sheaves of grain, the myths of autumn are often tied up to harvest and how we preserve and share what we've reaped. The edges of the land grow slightly fuzzy as the long spell of summer gives way to the dual energies of autumn's loosening (cutting down the grain) and tightening (bundling it up and storing it away). After the seemingly unending youth of summer we find ourselves in the middle age of autumn, hopefully a little wiser, with a lot of life already passed but a lot yet to live. We've tested summer's theories, explored our worlds in both practical and idealistic ways, and through our triumphs, tribulations, and grand mistakes, learned a thing or two about what living and dying may mean. Mostly, though, autumn shows us just how little we do know and how much there is still to learn.

Summer's fire transforms into the cool earth and air energy of autumn, guiding us to plant allies for brain health, herbal tonics to tone and clear airways, and gentle treatments for aches and pains arising with damper weather. Equinoxes are turning points, and while the spring equinox draws life upward and outward, the autumn equinox draws energy downward and inward, reconsidering what felt so certain under summer's glow. Autumn is excellent for making and stocking up remedies that protect our vitality, especially those blends that safeguard against common colds and illnesses. In traditional western herbalism, autumn is a time of fire meeting earth, drawing us into a season of structured stability as the fires of summer settle into a fixed and earthy form. The season is also a period of archetypal middle age, the compass direction west, and the fully ripened energy of the full moon. The call of earth draws us inward, using our energetic muscles to ground and center, exploring the edges of what feels familiar and strange, naming and embracing what it is that we would build a home for.

How will the shelter of summer stand as autumn tests the edges of what we've built?

**Joyful Summer, Golden Autumn Breathwork**

*For this breathwork I like to stand, but choose the position most comfortable for you. It can be extra magickal to do this leaning against a tree, large rock, or earthwork. Begin by taking a few gentle, centering breaths to find your rhythm. On the next exhalation, let your breath out slowly through your mouth. After a few rounds of breathing in through your nose and out through your mouth, try to make your exhalation last for as long as is comfortable and longer than your inhalation. Then at the end of every inhalation, pause and tense your whole or part of your body for a brief moment, followed by a long exhalation relaxing your body. Repeat this cycle of breath, tension, and relaxation until you feel a general state of relaxation come over you, like drifting or floating (which can seem extra secure if leaning against a tree or something else). Let yourself be held by the earth around you, gently releasing into autumn's embrace. End your breathwork session with some slow movement, allowing this feeling of relaxation to flow into all parts of your being.*

## The Gifts of Autumn

### *Boundaries*

Autumn holds the power of boundaries, of the edges between field and forest, river and valley, city blocks, suburban sprawl, and rural towns, as well as all those liminal spaces we hold within us and the dizzying array of social, cultural, and institutional partitions we encounter throughout our lives. Every act of healing is in some way boundary work, whether establishing a new boundary, renewing an already known boundary, or releasing an old boundary. Sometimes boundary



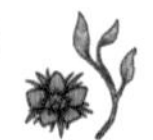

work is similar to a small repair, the emotional equivalent of patching up a tiny hole in a sweater with a bit of spare yarn. Other times we're digging up stones and building a wall or growing a hedge from seed. Whether you're studying to become a practicing herbalist or just want some familiarity with plants to help yourself and maybe some family and friends, exploring and understanding your internal boundaries, those of your practice, and those of the people you are in relationship with are part of the work.

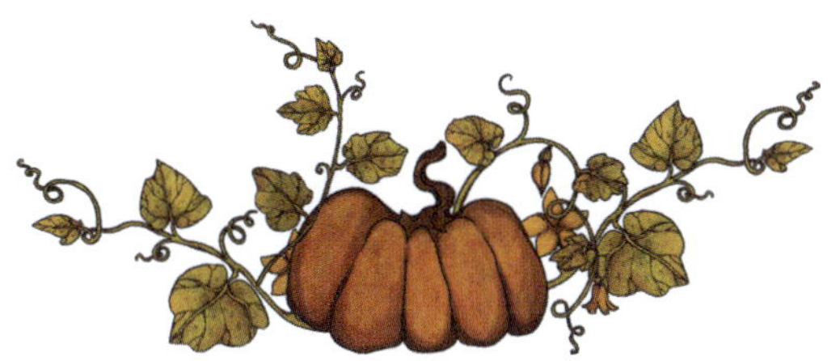

There are all sorts of interesting boundaries to observe on the land I live with. Few are hard and fixed; most represent a diversity of life around the edges; and many change throughout the seasons, days, and hours. I'm particularly attuned to limits of sun and shadow when it comes to the cycles of life and growth in the garden—having to plant seedlings, for example, to get enough winter light to thrive and survive any late season frosts but be covered by the shade of older plants to protect from the possibility of an overpowering mid-spring sun. Early autumn, though still warm, brings more and more shade and shadow to the garden and to city streets; the sun has changed its sky path, pulled down low by the equinox after months of its slow and long broad-chested saunter above us. The growing shadows likewise pull us to the boundary lands between the light and dark half of the year, pausing growth, bringing harvest and life-generating decay, and drawing energy earthward after months of stretching skyward. We test the boundaries of the shelters built during summer's long light, figuring out what will hold, what needs greater flexibility, and where we can continue to strengthen our edges.

Testing and having our boundaries tested, in nonviolent, often playful ways, are a normal process of development, when we get to say no and figure out what our yeses look like as we develop our sense of self. To resist autumn's boundaries is to go hungry for the protection and nourishment of self and our dignity that these boundaries protect. Boundaries are the shelters we carry with us, no matter what harsh emotional or physical environments we are crossing, and practices like gratitude are our sightlines, helping us chart our path. Every season of the year our life carries the power of boundaries, from the tender boundaries of spring in the form of new life breaking through to summer's shelter that protects us throughout the year and later winter's intangible boundaries of dream and possibility.

There are plenty of folks, though, who were led to ignore their inherent sense of secure boundary-creating—taught that this was a form of disobedience or developed from years in a state of exhaustion at having boundaries continuously tested or overrun. The experience of having a boundary violated or denied is dehumanizing, disconnecting us from our sense of self because it is by and through our boundaries that we experience who we are, what we want, and how we communicate with others. One of the most disheartening sorrows of modern life under global systems of exploitation is that we have all participated in these violations as standard practice for profit-making, and part of our work for social change and justice is learning how to navigate repair without falling into shame or despair. Recognizing missing boundaries and proceeding to establish and reinforce them through respectful relationships is at the heart of so much of what healing is, including reparative justice–centered healing. Thorny plants like Hawthorn (*Crataegus monogyna*), Rose (*Rosa* spp.), and Raspberry (*Rubus idaeus*) can be useful allies when we're learning to recognize and remember what feels right and secure.

The beginning and ending of seasons, both great and small, are the boundaries we all cyclically pass through—or sometimes we feel like they pass through us. As plant folk we are not only building a relationship to the autumn of the year, but learning to respect and be nourished by autumn's boundaries. As you explore your relationship to the land and its seasons, it can also be a fascinating process to explore the cultural seasons and boundaries you were raised with or surrounded by. There are also the boundaries of our internal cycles, from those of sleeping and waking, fertility, nervous system responses, and all our endless


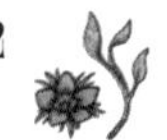

feelings. Autumn marks the line between growth and harvest, letting us know it's time to both speed up and gather and then slow down and take stock. To ignore autumn's boundary is to expect endless growth, plan for nothing, and find ourselves crossing over to winter unprepared.

Autumn, with its earthy energy, pulls us from the bright day of summer into the growing night of the dark half of the year, helping us to walk between our own worlds, feeling our way back home. As we continue to set boundaries—acknowledging first that we need them, honoring that they will change as we change and how they shape our life when we embrace them—we are also developing our skill for *feeling* our healing needs and what is and is not a path we're interested in taking. Long before I knew the word *somatic*, I was shaped by a magickal culture that recognized parts of us could get lost—little slivers of soul that go out and hide away, often as a result of a traumatic experience. Ritual and the celebration of seasonal sabbats are one way we feel and call all parts of ourselves back home. To call the soul home, you need to create a sacred boundary between the world outside and the world within so that a missing part feels supported and safe enough to be home again.

In my practice, I've come to recognize that a big part of boundary work is grappling with and embracing embodiment. Embodiment is an interesting intermingling of drawing inward, connecting between, and pulling outward. A few years back as I was going through my own journey of cultivating healthy boundaries, I noticed how many people seeking out herbalism, whether as clients or students, were looking for an embodied healing practice. All of us were drawn to plant ally work as one way to come back to our bodies and the land.

One reason herbalism is such a powerful embodiment practice is that most herbalists still rely on physically observable signs and the stories they hear to work with a client to understand what is happening. Sometimes the body speaks before the voice does, and as herbalists it's not our job to tell a person's story but to provide language through interpretation of the body's signs so that a client can shape their own narrative. Someone seeking support for chronic pain may have signs of Tension and Cold showing up as tight pain that moves toward the center of the body, culminating in poor circulation. In addition to drawing on herbs like warming relaxants, nervines, and circulatory tonics, we can offer our observations as opportunities to tell a story. Not only reflecting back a client's own words, but also describing pain we are observing as cold, hard, and stuck can create room for a client to explore what experiences, physical and emotional, may have brought on and continue to aggravate their pain. Then we can draw on the stories of the plants themselves, speaking on how a plant like Skullcap (*Scutellaria lateriflora*) has an incredible way of melting tension by helping us put our pain in perspective, shrinking down any anxiety or tension we hold about our pain.

As we establish boundaries, we begin to recognize where we begin and end, settling into deep embodiment of our earth-self and our connection to the land and community. Supporting our ability to feel embodied and connected to our inner and outer worlds is a process; it takes time to explore what feels good and honest enough for ourselves. If you're feeling overwhelmed about where to start exploring boundaries in your life, observing your cycles of sleep and rest can be one of the easier boundaries to spot in your internal explorations. Sometimes we have to seek out the places of dreams and memories to remember the shape of our land-body. Herbs like Mugwort (*Artemisia vulgaris*), Yarrow (*Achillea millefolium*), Holy Basil (*Ocimum tenuiflorum*), and Valerian (*Valeriana* spp.) can help us journey through these liminal spaces with ease.

Physically, as summer gives way to autumn and the weather begins to cool, our bodies start to cool and slow down, too. Summers are only growing longer and hotter in intensity, so we have to learn how to invest in shade and the shelter of rest. Summer shows us the importance of building, and autumn shows us how to expand. It's time to tend to the needs of the skin after a long season out of doors with vulneraries and astringents and turn to respiratory herbs to manage seasonal allergies, immunomodulators to build up our reserves and protect us from increasing exposure to colds, and joyful allies to alleviate seasonal sadness.

## *Expansion*

Every season holds the gift of expansion. Spring brings the energy of expanding growth, summer surrounds us in expansive heat and lush life, winter summons expansive quiet and slow darkness. I find autumn particularly infused with the energy of expansiveness, however, in no small part because harvest festivals reinforce our vast web of interdependence. There is a sense of maturity during autumn,

 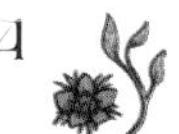 

when summer's youth is refined by the lessons of harvest. It's a time of year when, like in the spring, the boundaries between life and death feel tender and thin, porous and promising, as the boundaries of the land, of life, of communities, of access and opportunity, become more noticeable as thinner seasons arrive. Yet from the joy of the harvest table to life drawing in on itself as cold winds snap between increasingly bare branches and the sharp sides of skyscrapers, autumn's expansiveness thrums across the land.

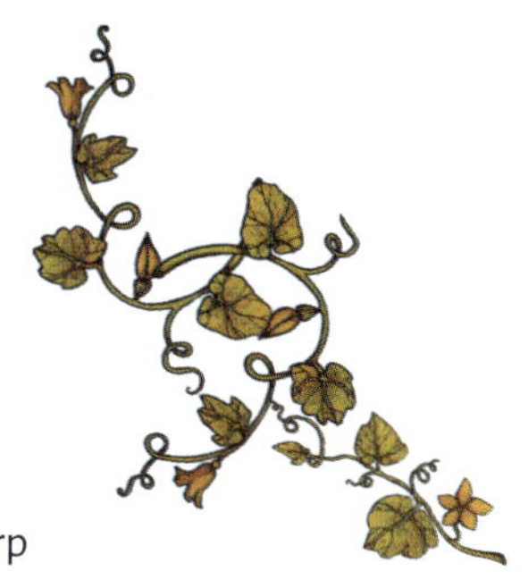

Expansiveness, the ability to extend beyond what seems possible, is at its steadiest and most daring when secure boundaries have been established. With resilient boundaries we have a better grasp of where we can journey beyond and the tools we need to carry to keep us grounded and centered as we go there. In other words, expansiveness should be a result of boundary work. I'm always amazed by what has been hidden by summer's green crown of foliage and flower becoming revealed again when leaves fall, fruit is gathered, and blossoms go to seed, leaving open windows and doorways to peer through like sudden portals to the otherworld. These otherworld openings, unnoticed within and around us, are what our expansiveness draws us toward. In autumn, I look out across my own inner landscape, over windswept valleys, beneath rock shelters, and between tide pools and shorelines to see where I am feeling most drawn to, where life feels big enough for living.

While spring carries the tender momentum of new life blossoming across the land, autumn's dance of boundaries and expansiveness draws energy down, inward, and through to the other side. While life expands in one season, death expands in another, and in autumn the land reflects to us lessons on limitations. Learning how to embrace seasons of death alongside seasons of life is one way many of us not only reclaim ancestral traditions, but release any fears of death keeping us tethered and tight while striving to preserve, create, and renew life-affirming traditions and sustainable practices. While death is a limitation all life on earth experiences, it is also a point of expansiveness, whether you believe in an afterlife or embrace the beautiful physics of our body's energy returning to the world around us. Many modern Pagans, myself included, observe autumn as the end of the year when the worlds of the living and the dead draw close for communion and exchange. As an herbalist, I'm always interested in a person's relationship to death, from honoring the harvest and transmutation of a living plant into an herbal remedy to their relationship to their own mortality. Peering into the unknowing depths of death—including when it might happen for us—is a practice of radical expansiveness that has the power to lead us back into a more loving and hopeful relationship with life.

In my practice, expansiveness marks a point of liminality, when what was and what might be on a person's healing path meet at the crossroads. It is a tender space and a bold one, too, where folks begin to imagine what a life beyond their current boundaries might feel like. Curiosity is an exceptionally useful tool for developing an expansive sense of self, of others, of dreams, and of healing. While I'm not interested at all in pushing anyone beyond their boundaries, I do love to point at little doorways and windows in a person's inner landscape and ask what might be through them. Often this is a combination of helping a person set appropriate containers of practice for their healing, such as protecting their boundaries of sleep and rest, and helping them generate a sense of possibility as they experience the results of their shelter-making (e.g., a protected sleep and rest cycle leading to more energy for doing things they love).

When someone is on a path of expansiveness, I want to make sure to connect them with all sorts of beautiful plant allies to support this time of regeneration. I often turn to gently energizing circulatory tonics like Turmeric (*Curcuma longa*), Rosemary (*Salvia rosmarinus*), and Hawthorn (*Crataegus monogyna*) to pull energy from wherever it is trapped in the body and bring it back into a healthy flow. Nervines with nootropic qualities like Ginkgo (*Ginkgo biloba*), Sage (*Salvia officinalis*), and Peppermint (*Mentha piperita*) are very helpful, since so much of the practice of expansion is tied to keeping our nervous system feeling supported while extending our perspectives and perceptions. Many of the herbs that can be harvested well into autumn, such as Rosemary (*Salvia rosmarinus*), Hawthorn (*Crataegus monogyna*), and Sage (*Salvia officinalis*), all carry qualities that support expansiveness, whether in energy, mental clarity, or openheartedness.

During autumn, I listen to the earth of my body and its changing and shifting boundaries. Where in my life does it feel easy to expand deeply? Where is their constraint or shallowness? I explore the edges of life, death, and rebirth,


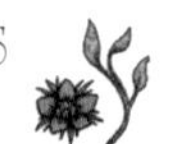

especially as I think of meeting with my ancestors at Samhain's feast and what it is I want to share with them considering the shape of my life during this past turning of the year. Most places I have lived have had very distinct autumn winds marking the end of summer and dramatically bringing in change. While spring winds carry our attention to the air of our respiratory system, autumn winds pull our focus to our largest organ and the process of oxygenation occurring through our skin. The strong earth energy of autumn creates an easy way to explore our skin's boundaries and expansiveness and support its health, since it is not only our organ most exposed to the environment around us but to all the beings we share the land with. I visit my inner landscape and observe what the land looks like on its surface from wild grasslands, tropical forests, and great swamps to desert plains, ice fields, high mountain meadows, and more. The land above can tell me a great deal about the land below, whether there is a diversity of microorganisms within the soil, deep water to draw from, good drainage and circulation, and the state of my mycelium nervous system.

Autumn is a season of earth, embodied simply through the harvest season, but also through the grand and complex, spanning endlessly diverse environments with varying levels of hospitality to life. Within Western esoteric tradition, earth is the element of the body, referring to both the physical and energetic bodies from our skeletal system to our skin to the energetic field moving within and around us. Our bodies are the physical home of our consciousness, shaped by millennia of life on our planet, yet incredibly finite. Working with our body and the energy of earth pulls us beyond the edges of what can be said or confined to words on a page and into a realm of deep feeling and interconnection. In traditional western herbalism, the seat of earth is the spleen, while modern western herbalism houses it in the musculoskeletal system. Earth shows up in all of the tissue states, but especially the solidifying energy of Cold and of Relaxation or the feeling of homeostasis. Herbs like Mullein (*Verbascum thapsus*), Plantain (*Plantago major, P. lanceolata*), Elder (*Sambucus nigra*), Hawthorn (*Crataegus monogyna*), Calendula (*Calendula officinalis*), Rose (*Rosa* spp.), and Red Clover (*Trifolium pratense*) all embody strong earth energy, helping to support the earth of our land-body.

The energy of earth brings the ability to feel and connect deeply with ourselves and other beings—skills essential to boundary-making and expansion. When we are struggling to process earth energy, we can find ourselves feeling ungrounded, overly exposed, exhausted, and low in energy. One of the best ways to support the earth of our inner landscape is by strengthening our capacity to connect and empathize while keeping our boundaries clear. Some of my favorite connecting and protecting activities include:

- Breathwork combined with gentle movement
- Skin-immersive activities like bathing, swimming, or water-based therapy
- Working with berries to strengthen, nourish, and beautify
- Reassessing what products you put on your skin
- Somatic forms of therapy, including dance, movement, art, and animal therapy
- Home and body blessings rituals for protection
- Making and using flower essences

## Autumn Inquiry

*What is my autumn story?*

*What does autumn feel, look, smell, and taste like in my body?*

*What does autumn feel, look, smell, and taste like in the land around me?*

*What is my experience of boundaries in my life and body?*

*What kind of boundaries do I find in the land and my communities?*

*How do boundaries shape my life?*

*How expansive does my life feel?*

*If I had enough in my life, what would I do?*

*If I were able to move freely in my life, where would I go?*



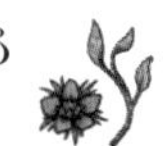

## Herbs for the Autumn Body

Within traditional western herbalism, autumn is a time of cold and damp earth softening the heat and dryness of summer. The long days of increase and growth are over, and now the land draws energy back into itself, including through processes of decay, so that over the long winter the soil can shelter the deep roots and fallen harvest seeds of a future spring's new growth. As summer retreats, the cooler weather brings dampness back to the land, pausing the evaporation of water by heat and absorption by hungry, growing plants. In traditional western herbalism, autumn represents the element of fire moving into earth and the sturdiness of middle age in the human life cycle. Supporting autumn energy within our apothecaries, we can turn to immunomodulating respiratory tonics to protect us from airborne viruses, expectorant herbs that clear out congestion, analgesics and anti-inflammatories for pain, as well as nootropics and circulatory tonics to support our maturing brains.

As summer's heat and dryness give way to the increasing damp of autumn, boundaries soften; the soil begins to renew with plant material falling back to earth; and the land exhales. The traditional Western energetic of Relaxation shows up in autumn's porousness and liminality, bringing with it gifts of rest and adaptability, being able to let go and flow freely. Relaxation can cause trouble for us when an imbalance leads to lack of tone, causing boundaries to collapse and overflow.

When the body becomes swamped with lack of Tension or boundaries and too much Relaxation, folks can experience a low-level fatigue that weakens the immune system, as well as imbalances of the body's fluids from fluid loss (e.g., excess sweating, heavy menstruation) to water retention. An interesting emotional aspect of excess Relaxation is that folks can feel confused about their identity and true needs, which can lead them to try to fit the expectations of those around them, unable to find their own sense of authentic self-expression. This state of excess Relaxation can bring on Tension, not only because of conditions such as high blood pressure, but also emotional and mental impact of a lack of control accompanied by the continuous loss a chronic Relaxation imbalance can bring. Astringent herbs like Dandelion (*Taraxacum officinale*), Yarrow (*Achillea millefolium*), and Raspberry Leaf (*Rubus idaeus*) can be very useful for the Relaxation tissue state, and adaptogens such as Holy Basil (*Ocimum tenuiflorum*), Ashwagandha (*Withania somnifera*), and Schisandra (*Schisandra chinensis*) can help the body relearn tone and bring out the beneficial adaptive nature of Relaxation.

As the season of middle age, when the body is at a midpoint between youth and elder, this can be a good time to start incorporating herbs supporting the longevity and adaptability of the aging body such as Sage (*Salvia officinalis*), Hawthorn (*Crataegus monogyna*), Lemon Balm (*Melissa officinalis*), Nettles (*Urtica dioica*), and Rose (*Rosa* spp.). Autumn is also a time of supporting our skin with vulnerary, emollient, and astringent herbs as well as our nervous system with nervous system tonics. It is also a powerful season to connect with stability and structure, including internal repair and reconnection with kind and gentle parental energy.

In Western esoteric tradition, earth is a symbol of ancestors and descendants, foundations and structures of life, death, and rebirth, and we can work with autumn's harvest and otherworldly energy to find the currents of healing and tradition that help us thrive. I often recommend folks work with the herbs of their ancestral lines to connect with autumnal energy, but you can also turn to our ancient plant allies such as Rose (*Rosa* spp.) and Ginkgo (*Ginkgo biloba*), which have been on our planet for millions of years, serving as collective plant ancestors. The land in autumn reflects the ways we create roots and legacies in our lives; we tend to the land not only for ourselves but for our living animal, plant, and elemental kin, as well as generations we won't ever know by name but who we can love right now as we care for their home.


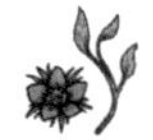

# Autumn Plant Allies

## Hawthorn

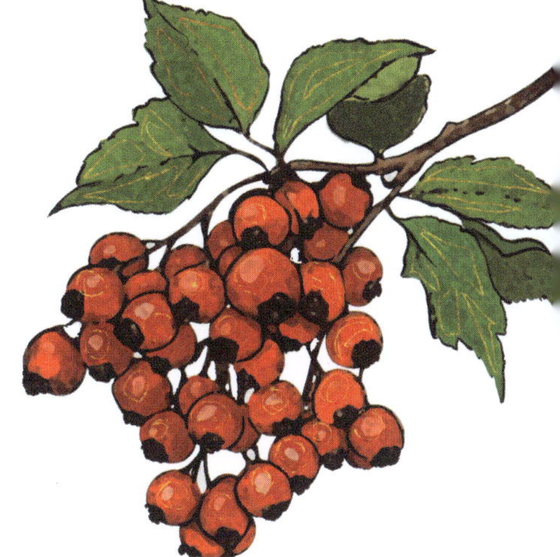

*(Crataegus monogyna)*

**Common + Folk Names:** May blossom or bush, whitethorn, chastity tree, bread and cheese tree, hagthorn

**Elements:** Fire, earth

**Zodiac Signs:** Embodies the energy of Leo and Scorpio. A remedy for Aries and Gemini.

**Planets:** Mars, Saturn, sun

**Moon Phase:** All moon phases

**Parts Used:** Leaf, flower, and berry

**Habitat:** Native to North America, Asia, and Europe

**Growing Conditions:** Full to partial sun in moist, well-drained soil. A common hedge and boundary plant.

**Collection:** Collect flowers and leaves in spring, berries in late summer and early fall.

**Flavor:** Sour and sweet

**Temperature:** Warm

**Moisture:** Dry

**Tissue States:** Cold, Stagnation

**Actions:** Cardiotonic, hypotensive, circulatory tonic, vasodilator, astringent, nervine, sedative, carminative, antispasmodic, amphoteric, anthelmintic, nutritive, diuretic, emollient, antioxidant, rejuvenative, adaptogenic, antibacterial, digestive, alterative, vulnerary, anti-inflammatory, mild expectorant

**Contraindications:** Generally considered safe, but use with caution with heart medications, bleeding disorders, and hypotension.

**Dosage:** Standard dosage. Hawthorn should be taken at least three months for full benefits.

Hawthorn is a plant of hedges and hinges, helping us navigate all the experiences of the heart, from its emotional needs to its physical health. It is an ally of the brokenhearted and those times when a wound has left us feeling shattered, vulnerable, or pulled apart. During these moments, Hawthorn arrives with bravehearted joy, unafraid to travel the shadowlands to find and mend what has been broken.

As a cardiac trophorestorative, Hawthorn brings the hardworking heart muscle back into balance after illness, prolonged stress, or the effects of aging. It is best used over a minimum of three months and gentle enough for all ages. Antioxidant-rich, Hawthorn prevents and reverses damage caused by free radicals as well as reducing oxidative stress on the capillary walls and improving circulation—helping to balance between Relaxation and Tension tissue states.[14] It should be considered in cases of palpitations and irregular heartbeat, angina, hardening arteries, heart enlargement from excessive exercise or overwork, hypertension, both low and high blood pressure, and too much cholesterol. Hawthorn can also be used for issues with blood vessels in general, including varicose veins, hemorrhoids, and ulcers. Hawthorn's blood pressure–stabilizing effect also settles the nervous system, improving cardiac function and creating a general state of ease in the body.

As I work with a lot of highly sensitive folks, I often turn to Hawthorn to help them heal the brokenheartedness arising from being told to "stop being so



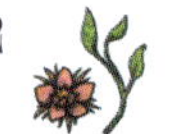

sensitive" or to "just get over it" in response to the enormity of their emotional experiences. Hawthorn protects our emotional vulnerability with its thorns, allowing us to open up to our vulnerability in a healing and restorative way. I love the language used by Judith Berger to describe it: "As guardian of the hinge, hawthorn wisely discerns the right timing for the wounded heart to open."[15]

Hawthorn is also for those who feel wild and overstimulated in their grief and heartbreak. It calms, soothes, and protects, which is what we need more than ever when we feel raw. Hawthorn can also be an aid for neurodiverse folks struggling with overstimulation, irritability, and restlessness—Hawthorn's calming energy supports the work of self-regulation.

In addition to heart-healing qualities, Hawthorn is a gentle diuretic, cleansing the lymph system, helping blood flow freely, and alleviating the Stagnation that can arise from a weak or overworked heart caused by excess stress. Hawthorn berries are chock-full of bioflavonoids, which improve collagen and strengthen joints and connective tissues. It also reduces inflammation throughout the body, helping to lower cholesterol and regulate blood pressure.

For the elderly, Hawthorn is especially well-suited for improving cardiovascular tone and reducing the possibility of angina attacks by dilating the arteries. It also reduces the buildup of fat in the liver and aorta as well as assists in the prevention, disintegration, and passage of urinary stones and gravel. In general, if there is a legacy of heart disease in the family, Hawthorn might be a good long-term ally for your preventative wellness plan. It also supports healthy circulatory tone for premenopausal and menopausal folks. While primarily a cardiotonic, Hawthorn functions as a tonic for stagnant digestion, when food is not properly digested, leading to symptoms of indigestion, diarrhea, and cramping.

Externally, the flowers can be used in facial steams and washes to improve complexion and reduce rosacea. Use the berries in gargles for sore throats and bleeding gums.

**Seasonal Uses**

When spring arrives, I add Hawthorn to tea blends to move from the relative quiet of winter to the busyness of spring, as it helps to gently cleanse the lymphs. In summer I add Hawthorn to all my heart-expanding blends. Hawthorn is especially useful in autumn as the weather changes and nights grow longer, steadying us even during the dark of the year. In winter I like to add Hawthorn to cold and flu blends when heart palpitations and indigestion are present.

**Magickal Uses**

Hawthorn's primary magickal use is for protection. Traditionally Hawthorn is hung in bundles above doorways and beds to guard against unwanted energy, lightning strikes, and illness. It has a strong association with the magick of the hedgerows, acting as a boundary between our world and the otherworld, and the Good Folk are said to meet beneath the Hawthorn tree, making it useful for trancework. Add the thorns to charms of protection to safeguard you on your journeys throughout all the worlds.

Hawthorn is associated with both fertility and death, tying it to Beltane and Samhain. Incorporate the blossoms into your Beltane magick, including fertility spells and handfasting blessings, and bathe your face with the dew from Hawthorn on Beltane morning for a year of beauty. Add the berries and thorns to your Samhain rites to travel safely to meet your ancestors in thin places.

**The Hawthorn Personality**

The brokenhearted and grieving have a special place in the Hawthorn circle, as the herb opens the heart after a period of despair. Hawthorn is an ally for those who grieve for the world, with many sensing injustice from a very early age. As children, Hawthorn folk can appear more like changelings than a fully human child. Their profound grief can create a wild restlessness in their life, whereby they struggle to feel settled at home and work or in their relationships. Sometimes they are punished for the everyday acts of an energetic child and disdained for their enthusiasm—they close up their heart to protect it from the hostility of a world preferring they sit quietly at a desk for hours instead of dance around in joy. Hawthorn reopens the heart and helps folks connect with their resiliency and capacity to let go of stories that have harmed them and remain protected as they begin to express themselves and all their energy with pride and intention. When Hawthorn folk are in their power, they possess an ability to tap into calm amid life's tumultuousness, extending that gift to others and helping folks find the tools to express themselves honestly and beautifully.


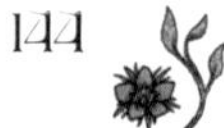

# Mullein

*(Verbascum thapsus)*

**Common + Folk Names:** Hag's tapers, beggar's blanket, graveyard dust, candlewick, Jupiter's staff, torches, velvet dock, witch's candle, lungwort, shepherd's staff, verbasco, nookaadiziiganzh

**Elements:** Earth, water

**Zodiac Signs:** Embodies the energy of Capricorn. A remedy for Taurus, Gemini, and Leo.

**Planet:** Saturn

**Moon Phase:** Waning quarter moon

**Parts Used:** Leaf, flower, root

**Habitat:** Native to Eurasia and North Africa but naturalized throughout North America

**Growing Conditions:** Grows in waste areas and roadsides. Likes full sun and well-drained soil.

**Collection:** Collect the flowers and leaves from second-year and older plants, roots in the fall.

**Flavor:** Pungent, slightly bitter

**Temperature:** Cool

**Moisture:** Moist

**Tissue States:** Stagnation, Dryness

**Actions:** Alterative, anodyne, antibacterial, antihistamine, anti-inflammatory, antiseptic, antispasmodic, antiviral, astringent, decongestant, demulcent, diuretic, emollient, expectorant, pectoral, vulnerary. *Flower:* Analgesic, anti-inflammatory, antispasmodic, demulcent, emollient, mucilaginous, nervine, sedative. *Root:* Anti-inflammatory, antispasmodic, anodyne, diuretic, nervine.

**Contraindications:** Considered generally safe

**Dosage:** Standard dosage

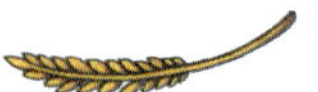

Mullein is a great ally for clearing phlegm from the system, reducing inflammation, and protecting against infection. It's excellent for clearing out chronic, long-standing coughs, especially dry and spasmodic coughs, and can help with a number of respiratory complaints, from bronchitis to asthma to general lung weakness. Mullein also has a long history as a remedy for tuberculosis, whooping cough, and pleurisy. Indications for Mullein include a chesty, chronic cough that worsens when lying down and has resulted from or contributed to adrenal stress, especially after long bouts of illness. Add it to your cold and flu blends with Elder (*Sambucus nigra*) and Peppermint (*Mentha piperita*) for a lung-opening, immunostimulating blend.

As a decongestant, Mullein is good for allergies such as hay fever, clearing phlegm and relieving pain. In her *Physica*, Hildegard von Bingen recommended Mullein for "one who is hoarse or has a pain in his chest," suggesting they combine the herb with Fennel (*Foeniculum vulgare*) in a medicinal wine.[16] Use also for asthma (especially with heat and aggravation) and general chest infections. Mullein's immunostimulating qualities mean it is not only good for cold and flu season, but can work for someone struggling with chronic viral infections.

As a moistening diuretic, Mullein soothes an inflamed urinary system and helps with the release of urine. Mullein is also well-suited for cases of edema and water retention as well as arthritis, rheumatism, gout, UTIs, and cystitis. As a digestive tonic, Mullein is a mild bitter that relieves indigestion, especially with damp and stagnant digestion, and can alleviate the pain of peptic ulcers.

Mullein's analgesic qualities can be applied for nerve pain, and it combines well with other pain-relieving nervines such as Skullcap (*Scutellaria lateriflora*) and St. Joan's Wort (*Hypericum perforatum*). Use internally as a tea or tincture as well as externally as an herbal oil for neuralgia and especially nerve pain in the hands and feet. In particular, the root can be used in cases of Bell's palsy and facial nerve pain. Mullein loosens up stiff joints and tense connective tissue.

Topically, the mucilaginous Mullein is excellent for dry skin conditions and as a healing compress or salve for boils, bruises, inflammation, hemorrhoids, eczema, sciatica, and joint pain. Use in a steam for lung conditions like asthma, bronchitis, and other respiratory imbalances already described. Cree and Métis herbalist Mary Siisip Geniusz recommends following a Mullein herbal steam with a cup of Yarrow (*Achillea millefolium*) tea in bed to clear the head and chest.[17] Mullein is used similarly as a smoking herb as well as an aid in weaning off tobacco. Mullein is helpful in cases of bulging discs and bone-setting. It assists in skin repair after a wound, burn, sore, and ulcer and can be used for skin infections, too.

A compress of the leaves is excellent for alleviating the pain of swollen joints, sore muscles, swollen glands, eczema, and headaches. For sprains, gather up fresh Sage (*Salvia officinalis*) and Mullein leaves, gently bruise them, and wrap them around the sprained joint. Create a gargle of the tea or extract for laryngitis, swollen gums, and tonsillitis. Mullein and Garlic ear oil is a trusted remedy for ear infections—I always keep a small bottle of this in my home apothecary just for that reason.

### Seasonal Uses

In spring I use Mullein to relieve any lingering winter coughs or chest congestion, as well as protect against seasonal allergies. Summer is full of Mullein harvests to store for the rest of the year, and I frequently use the fresh leaves for sprains, strains, and all sort of pain. In the autumn I turn to Mullein as a respiratory tonic and antihistamine to keep my respiratory system strong. For winter, Mullein is a great addition to cold-care blends for coughs and to strengthen the immune system.

### Magickal Uses

The long thick stems are sometimes referred to as hag's tapers (dried stalks dipped in wax or fat will burn as a somewhat messy candle) as they are associated with the magickal workings of witchfolk. So it is no surprise Mullein is a plant long associated with the working of hags or those women, often elders, who seem dangerously uncontrollable or unpalatable to dominant power systems. Use Mullein in your magickal rites to honor your hag and witch ancestors.

Mullein is associated with protection and travelers. You can tuck the leaves into your shoe for added comfort and protection on your journeys. Use for general protection spells and specifically against the Night Mare, who brings us unwanted night visions. The powdered herb can be a substitute for graveyard dust in spells and charms. Burn Mullein in your Midsummer bonfire for protection and gather the ashes to use in protection charms.

### The Mullein Personality

The Mullein person has something to get off their chest, which can sometimes manifest as chronic respiratory infections and a barking cough that won't allow them to get a clear word out. Their adrenals are often run-down, and mornings—just as they are getting out of bed—can be a difficult time for them physically and emotionally. Often, Mullein folk come off as dried out, but this may be because all of their waters have pooled deep in the body. With this reservoir of unexpressed truth, they are stewing—sometimes even bubbling over. They need to learn how to light their torch, even if the words that come aren't perfectly illuminating or up to their standards. Mullein folk can be confused about what they stand for because they have been so focused on "correct" social customs and traditions but yearn to step out of line. Mullein will help them to become honest with themselves and release these stagnant patterns of seeking external authority so that they can speak their own words freely. When living in their power, Mullein folk have an incredible ability to point out the ways we have been shaped by cultural norms doing us more harm than good and then, with their torches brightly lit, can illuminate the path toward the bonfires of connection, storytelling, and dancing free.



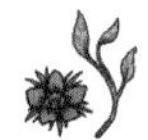

# Plantain

*(Plantago major, P. lanceolata)*

**Common + Folk Names:** Ribwort, cuckoo's bread, Englishman's foot, leaf of Patrick, ripplegrass, snakebite, snakeweed, waybread, weybroed, wegbrāde, whiteman's footsteps, ginebigowashk

**Element:** Earth

**Zodiac Signs:** Embodies the energy of Taurus, Libra, and Capricorn. A remedy for Leo and Aquarius.

**Planet:** Venus

**Moon Phase:** Full moon

**Parts Used:** Leaf (primarily), seed (occasionally)

**Habitat:** Widely naturalized, including in heavily urbanized areas

**Growing Conditions:** Grows in all types of soil, preferring part to full sun

**Collection:** Harvest leaves throughout spring and summer. Harvest seeds at the end of summer, early autumn.

**Flavor:** Sweet, salty, bitter

**Temperature:** Cool

**Moisture:** Dry

**Tissue States:** Heat, Stagnation, Relaxation

**Actions:** *Leaf:* Alterative, antibacterial, anti-inflammatory, antiseptic, antispasmodic, anthelmintic, anitvenomous, astringent, expectorant, decongestant, demulcent, deobstruent, depurative, diuretic, febrifuge, hemostatic, ophthalmic, mucilaginous, refrigerant, restorative, vulnerary. *Seed:* Demulcent, fiber laxative, emollient.

**Contraindications:** Generally regarded as safe, but herbalist Anne McIntyre suggests caution with lithium and carbamazepine (as Plantain may reduce effectiveness) and avoid with warfarin and anticoagulants.

**Dosage:** Standard dosage

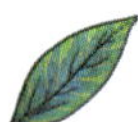

To get to know Plantain, let's start with a thousand-year-old herbal charm against poison coming to us through the Anglo-Saxon herbal tradition, one of the wisdom streams of traditional western herbalism. The Nine Herbs Charm was recorded in *The Lacnunga* sometime between the 9th and 10th centuries as a salve against poison. In it Plantain—called *Wegbrāde* in the dialect of the time or Waybread in modern English—is described as a plant protecting against poisons and evil:

> *And you, Waybread, mother of plants*
> *open to the east, mighty within,*
> *carts ran over you, ladies rode over you,*
> *brides cried over you, bulls snorted over you,*
> *you withstood them all and you were crushed,*
> *so may you withstand the poison and infection*
> *and the evil that travels round the land.*[18]

Like many herbal students trained in the Western tradition, I first learned about Plantain as an invaluable salve, and when I encountered the Nine Herbs Charm a few years later, I was delighted to see the roots in old tradition passed down in one form or another through the ages. This tale of survival speaks to a practical tenacity among the healing gifts of Plantain. It is a beautiful remedy that can show up in the toughest of places to aid folks in hard situations.

Plantain is known primarily for two healing gifts: It is a powerful drawing agent and a diuretic that regulates fluids, acting as a sort of trophorestorative for the fluid systems of the body. It is helpful in cases of urinary tract infections and bed-wetting, it alleviates menorrhagia, and it regulates fluid, from expelling excess mucus to bringing moisture to dried-out body systems (including the skin). Plantain can also be used as a tonic for the lymphatic system. English herbalist Thomas Bartram describes Plantain as a "neuralgic remedy of the highest order" and recommends using the tincture topically by "paint[ing] over painful areas of shingles, etc."[19] A Plantain and Mullein (*Verbascum thapsus*) salve or liniment can be used as a compress on the back and along the spine for pain relief as well as anywhere else on the body needing support.

For colds and fevers, Plantain can help to reduce fevers, alleviate sore throats, and reduce congestion. In general, Plantain is an ally for inflammation, bringing cooling energy to all body systems, including overheated conditions of the stomach and intestines such as gastritis and IBS. Use Plantain during allergy season to reduce inflammation and alleviate hay fever, as well as resolve respiratory infections. Plantain is also an important ally for those living in areas affected by fires. During fire season, I turn to herbs like Plantain for healing tissue and restoring the lungs after inhaling the particulate matter carried in smoke, blending it with herbs like Mullein (*Verbascum thapsus*) and Hyssop Leaf (*Hyssopus officinalis*) in tincture form.

Topically, Plantain is a powerful skin remedy for wound care, healing damaged tissue, and alleviating pain. If Plantain is growing nearby when you or someone else is stung by a bee or other insect, crush up a Plantain leaf and apply it to the bite for pain relief and reduction of swelling. Plantain can be drunk as a tea and used internally as a douche for vaginal yeast infections. Herbalist Deb Soule recommends pouring hot water over the seeds to make a gel that can be strained and used to soothe inflamed labia.[20]

Take Plantain internally and use as an external wash for cases of acne. Use as a gargle for tooth and gum complaints, as a hair rinse for dandruff, and as a wash for irritated skin, including eczema. The plant can also be used as an eye rinse for irritated eyes (e.g., in the case of fire or allergy season) and conjunctivitis. Similar to Mullein (*Verbascum thapsus*), Plantain can relieve foot weariness.

### Seasonal Uses

A great addition to cleansing spring tonics, I use Plantain to clear congestion and reduce inflammation. Summer is a busy time of Plantain harvest, for drying, powdering, tincturing, and salve-making, and I make sure to keep the tincture on hand to deal with any excessive environmental pollution. In autumn, Plantain is a frequent addition to antihistamine remedies and blends for restoring skin health after a long season outdoors. For winter, Plantain is a welcome ingredient in most cold-care blends for alleviating pain and inflammation.

### Magickal Uses

As a traditional remedy for snakebite, Plantain is associated with the magick of snakes and can be used in place of or to represent snake skin and parts in spells and rituals. It is said to remove weariness, and Scott Cunningham notes a tradition of wrapping Plantain around the head with red wool to alleviate headache.[21]

### The Plantain Personality

Just as Plantain can spend a lot of time underfoot, so, too, can Plantain folks suffer from feeling like they are under the energy of everyone around them. Sometimes this manifests as feeling oppressed and disempowered in their relationships—whether romantic, familial, social, professional—because they seem to be (and often are) overlooked and underappreciated. They find themselves expected to always be there but never acknowledged for how much effort that takes—how exhausting! Sometimes this creates an overactive fawning response, other times a martyr complex, but both are simply coping mechanisms that can be transformed with proper therapeutic support and healing relationships. A Venusian plant, Plantain helps folks to step into their beauty, to be seen and appreciated, while also seeing and loving themselves. Plantain helps folks examine patterns of relating to themselves and others that need readjusting or dissolving altogether, for it is a plant that knows how to pull out whatever is poisoning our well of wisdom. When dwelling in their power, Plantain folks are tenaciously present, powerful, and fearless in their endeavors to help themselves and others feel held and whole.


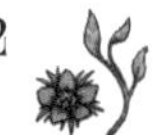

# The Autumn Apothecary

## Embodied Wisdom: Herbs for the Musculoskeletal System

### *Herbal Actions*

*Analgesics, anti-inflammatories, and antioxidant-rich herbs*

Aging is a gift of expansion and contraction, reflected back at us through our body, especially in our musculoskeletal system. As we get older, it's good to be familiar with a variety of herbs that support our structural body, from our skeleton and cartilage to our muscles, ligaments, tendons, joints, and connective tissues. For more specific recommendations for conditions like arthritis and chronic pain, see the Rain Is Coming (page 155) section.

**Ashwagandha (*Withania somnifera*):** My favorite topical treatment for muscle health for all ages is a simple herbal oil made of Ashwagandha, but it can also be taken internally as a powder, tincture, and so forth. Use after athletic performance, recovering from illness, or whenever you're in pain. Indications include tight pain and headaches, general fatigue including muscle weakness, and swelling.

**Burdock (*Arctium lappa*):** Great for rebuilding resilience in the body after a period of illness or fatigue, Burdock is a nutritive that acts as a restorative tonic for undernourished body systems, including supporting the health of the aging body. Indications include signs of ineffective circulation, such as redness of the joints, increased sensitivity to environmental pollutants, and general fatigue.

**Myrrh (*Commiphora molmol*):** Myrrh is a powerful source of antioxidants, helping to restore life and energy to overworked body systems, including the musculoskeletal system. A great preventative against degenerative diseases, indications include joint pain, arthritis, amenorrhea and dysmenorrhea, swollen lymph nodes, and fatigue.

**Red Clover (*Trifolium pratense*):** A good example of a vitamin- and mineral-rich herb that protects bone from conditions like osteoporosis, Red Clover is great to incorporate into regular rotation for daily teas and tonics. Indications include inflammation, lymphatic congestion and swelling, cramps, and fatigue.

**Rosemary (*Salvia rosmarinus*):** Rosemary moves energy throughout the body, improving mobility and energy. The herb can be used internally as a tea and extract as well as externally as a compress, herbal oil, bath, and liniment. Indications include conditions of stagnation, low energy and mood, headaches, sciatica, and neuralgia.

## Tending the Soul Shrine: Supporting the Health & Beauty of Our Skin

### *Herbal Actions*

*Vulneraries, astringents, and nervines*

While I've already written about more first-aid and post-sun exposure treatments for the skin in the summer apothecary, the following plant allies are great at supporting general skin health and radiance and protecting our skin as the weather turns cooler.

**Calendula (*Calendula officinalis*):** Calendula is one of my favorite end-of-summer, start-of-autumn herbal oils to use on my skin. Applying a Calendula herbal oil from my spring harvest feels like infusing my skin with the last bit of summer's heat before I welcome the much anticipated coolness of autumn and cold of winter. It's a great plant ally in all its forms (herbal oil, flower for tea, and flower essence) for those struggling with sadness at the change from the light to the dark half of the year. Indications include wounds and varicosities, sun- and windburn, and dull skin.

**Chamomile (*Matricaria chamomilla*):** This is a great remedy for "cranky" skin, including conditions like eczema, psoriasis, and dandruff. Indications include inflammation and overly sensitive skin, acne, and redness.

**Rose (*Rosa* spp.):** My absolute favorite herb for skin wellness, I love Rose in all of its forms. Rose hydrosol is a wonderful way to clean and tone the skin, while rosehip oil is a nutrient-rich serum to help the skin glow and Rose added to teas protects against free radicals. Indications include red and irritated skin, such as rashes and acne-prone skin, but in general, Rose is a good tonic herb for most skin types.

**Turmeric (*Curcuma longa*):** I love Turmeric for its ability to protect the skin against environmental stress and pollution as well as address issues like eczema, acne, and inflammation. Turmeric also reduces sensory overwhelm in our environments, starting from the skin down, by helping with inner body system regulation (e.g., it's easier to feel less irritated and overwhelmed by sound pollution when you're not also having to deal with a slow digestive system causing cramping and discomfort). Indications include extrasensitive skin and irritated skin, dullness, scarring, and dryness.

## Rain Is Coming: Managing Arthritis & Other Chronic Pain

### *Herbal Actions*

*Anti-inflammatories, analgesics, and digestives/stomachics*

Whether from arthritis or an old injury, sometimes when the weather becomes cooler and damper, discomfort and pain can increase. As with all herbal recommendations, plant remedies for the musculoskeletal system, which is complex and a common place to experience pain, should be complemented with movement-based and bodywork therapies, nourishing food practices, and mental health support. The following plants provide much needed pain relief so you can enjoy sweater weather better.

**Black Cohosh (*Actaea racemosa*):** A good herb for those struggling with chronic pain and its associated emotional pain, Black Cohosh can be a great choice for folks who have a history of trauma leading to their chronic pain, alleviating the tension that trauma can create in our lives. Indications include sciatica, neuralgia, fibromyalgia, a history of trauma, a feeling of hopelessness, muscle tightness, pain that worsens with movement, and a general feeling of constriction.

**Cramp Bark (*Viburnum opulus*):** While alleviating uterine cramping is where Cramp Bark really excels, it can also be employed for other muscle cramps and spasms, including lower back pain. (Consider combining with *Taraxacum officinale* or *Verbascum thapsus* when you're also trying to strengthen the back or with *Hypericum perforatum* if there is nerve pain or discomfort.) You can include Cramp Bark in your post-workout blends to alleviate and prevent muscle pain and fatigue. Indications include conditions of excess stagnation, intestinal and stomach cramps, cramping caused by IBS, and general fatigue.

**Feverfew (*Tanacetum parthenium*):** A great migraine preventative tonic, especially when taken in small doses over an extended period of time, Feverfew can also be used for rheumatoid arthritis and inflamed, painful skin conditions like dermatitis. Indications include tooth pain, muscle and joint pain, and mild depression.

**Meadowsweet (*Filipendula ulmaria*):** Meadowsweet is a powerful tonic for heat in the body from arthritic inflammation, fever, heartburn, or similarly overheated conditions. Pain and indigestion are frequently connected, which is why Meadowsweet's qualities as a digestive tonic make it valuable in pain care. Indications include indigestion, especially nausea leading to heartburn, headaches caused by pain elsewhere in the body, and connective tissue weakness.

**Turmeric (*Curcuma longa*):** *Haldi doodh*, or golden milk, is my favorite daily anti-inflammatory remedy, and Turmeric is the main ingredient. When making or purchasing Turmeric, you want to get a variety high in *curcumin*, which is what makes Turmeric such a beautiful anti-inflammatory. Make sure to add Black Pepper to the mix so that the *curcumin* becomes more bioavailable. Turmeric can be used internally and externally for pain. Indications include rheumatoid arthritis and gout, IBS, and weakened immunity.

**Vervain (*Verbena officinalis, V. hastata*):** A good remedy for pain caused by stress leading to excess tension, including migraine headaches (combine with *Betonica officinalis*). Indications include shoulder and neck tension, inflexibility of body and mentality, and sore throat.

**White Willow Bark (*Salix alba*):** Willow's inner bark contains salicin, which relieves fever, pain, and inflammation. As a cooling, anti-inflammatory herb, Willow can

be used internally and externally to clear heat from conditions such as rheumatoid arthritis, hot flashes, and headaches exacerbated by heat. White Willow Bark is great for reducing pain and improving mobility, helping in cases of backache, migraines, and general soreness. It combines well with Meadowsweet for reduction of rheumatic pain as well as conditions such as fibromyalgia. Indications include conditions of excess Heat, headaches, gout, arthritis, and backache.

**Wood Betony (*Betonica officinalis*):** If your chronic pain is mostly located above the shoulders, Wood Betony might be a good ally. It addresses general pain but is especially prized for headaches and migraines as well as facial pain. Indications include racing thoughts, anxiety, general fatigue, tension, and the type of chronic pain that flares up with stress.

## Damp & Dust & Runny Noses: Addressing Autumn Allergies

### *Herbal Actions*

*Anti-inflammatory, antihistamine, anticatarrhal, and respiratory tonics*

For my full list of recommendations for seasonal allergies, see the spring apothecary, but I've listed a few favorite autumn allergy plant allies here.

**Garlic (*Allium sativum*):** A wonderfully grounding and delicious plant to work with, Garlic connects us with the earthy energy of autumn while helping to regulate respiratory function. Indications include general allergies, respiratory weakness, asthma, and low immunity.

**Marshmallow (*Althea officinalis*):** Autumn brings cooler temperatures but holds on to summer's dryness, which can be extra irritating for everything from the skin to the respiratory system. Marshmallow is moistening and soothing, improving vitality while alleviating allergies. Indications include signs of acidity and inflammation, dry coughs, and rough, dry skin.

**Plantain (*Plantago major, P. lanceolata*):** I like to add Plantain to allergy blends to help bodies pass the common environmental allergens from dust, dander, mold, and pollen. Indications include congestion, brain fog, runny nose, and sore throats.

## Everything in Balance: Herbs for the Hormonal System

### *Herbal Actions*

*Hormonal tonics, nervines, adaptogens, and circulatory tonics*

Working in close relationship to the nervous system (see The Singing Land, page 70), the endocrine system manages hormonal regulation throughout the body through the thyroid, parathyroid, pituitary, and adrenal glands, as well as the pancreas, ovaries, and testes. The following herbs support general hormonal health, but for more specific recommendations for menstrual health check out The Lunar Body section (page 162) as well as hormonal sections in the summer and winter apothecaries.

**Ashwagandha (*Withania somnifera*):** A great hormonal regulator, especially if there are issues with the internal and external reproductive organs. Indications include chronic pain such as from fibromyalgia, menstrual dysregulation, chronic fatigue, impotence, prostate problems, and nervous exhaustion.

**Bacopa (*Bacopa monnieri*):** If hormonal dysregulation has been brought on by stress, calming but revitalizing Bacopa might be a good remedy. Indications include stress-related skin conditions, pain and swelling, low energy, anxiety, and agitation.

**Hawthorn (*Crataegus monogyna*):** When the hormonal system is overstimulated leading to excess tension, consider Hawthorn. Indications include restlessness, heart palpitations, confusion and lack of focus, recovering from heartbreak, and feeling overstimulated because of grief.

**Holy Basil (*Ocimum tenuiflorum*):** A great overall tonic for the hormonal system, Holy Basil regulates energy throughout all body systems, bringing us into a state of homeostasis. Indications include brain fog, infertility, menstrual dysregulation, low immunity, mild depression, and insomnia.


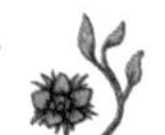

**Milky Oat (*Avena sativa*):** A powerful nervine, Milky Oat also helps restore an exhausted endocrine system. Indications include nervous exhaustion, physical weakness, burnout, poor memory and concentration, and stress ranging from acute anxiety to panic attacks.

## An Ounce of Prevention: Preventing Cold & Flu

### *Herbal Actions*

*Immunomodulators, anti-inflammatories, and nervines*

A lot of herbal medicine is focused on preventative measures and the ways we can incorporate healing plants into our daily life. While I look at plant allies for the common cold and the flu in the winter apothecary, the following recommendations are for herbs as preventative tonics to strengthen and regulate immunity.

**Elder (*Sambucus nigra*):** As summer ends and autumn begins, I make some Elderberry syrup, and it becomes a staple remedy in our household. Elder works to prevent colds and influenza but also shortens the duration if you happen to catch either. Indications include red, dry skin, slow digestion and elimination, low immunity, and general congestion.

**Milky Oat (*Avena sativa*):** As stress is the underlying reason for many diseases and discomforts, working with a friendly nervine like Milky Oat on a regular basis is one of the best measures you can adopt. Milky Oat is one of my favorite nervines and best taken over an extended period (six months and longer). Indications include feeling dried out internally and externally, mild depression, anxiety, and exhaustion.

**Shatavari (*Asparagus racemosus*):** A highly valued restorative tonic within Ayurvedic tradition, Shatavari is regarded as a panacea. Similar to Milky Oat as a nervine, Shatavari is more energizing, helping to modulate the immune system and prevent infection. Indications include body system dysregulation from hormonal issues (e.g., irregular menstruation, hair loss, or hormonal acne); signs of overheated digestion, including diarrhea; and general fatigue.

**Thyme (*Thymus vulgaris*):** A simple kitchen remedy, Thyme strengthens the immune system without overstimulating it. Indications include signs of stagnation like congestion and a slow metabolism, feelings of ungroundedness, and brain fog.

## The Growing Shadow: Alleviating the Symptoms of Seasonal Sadness

### *Herbal Actions*

*Nervines, antidepressants, and anxiolytics*

While feeling melancholic from time to time is a normal part of life, including when the seasons change from the bright half to the dark half of the year, when you're experiencing persistent sadness during autumn and winter it's time to seek support. While I've listed some plants allies for those affected by seasonal sadness, they are meant to be used *alongside* other healing modalities like therapy, bodywork, and other forms of medicine. Hopefully, as plants are prone to do when we open up to their wisdom, they'll guide you to the places and spaces you need to be to find wellness throughout the year.

One style of remedy I recommend for folks seeking to alleviate their seasonal depression is anything that cultivates a sense of comfort. What a comforting remedy is will be different for everyone, but for me, a warm glass of oat milk blended with powdered herbs and spices is the most comforting. You might find your comforting remedy in childhood memories (e.g., the scent of Peppermint always makes you feel taken care of because of the menthol rubs you got as a child) or in ancestral and/or cultural traditions that may or may not have been passed down to you. Becoming curious about your comfort or anything else that piques your interest is one way to guard against and alleviate some of the discomfort of seasonal sadness, so I encourage you to give it a try.

**Ashwagandha (*Withania somnifera*):** As the evenings grow cold, I love preparing a warm cup of Ashwagandha milk before bed. Ashwagandha is a nervous system restorative, meaning it helps to repair an exhausted, overwhelmed, and overworked nervous system. It's a lovely ally to work with over an extended period of time and a good option if you find other adaptogenic herbs too overstimulating to your system. Indications include mental and physical fatigue, sadness brought on by overwork and exhaustion, and expecting too much of yourself.

**Holy Basil (*Ocimum tenuiflorum*):** A sturdy friend during hard times, Holy Basil is a well-loved restorative within Ayurvedic tradition, uplifting the spirit, relieving anxiety, and easing depression. Consider combining with herbs like Ashwagandha (*Withania somnifera*) and Rose (*Rosa* spp.) for alleviating seasonal sadness. Indications include excess cold conditions, insomnia, difficulty sliding into a meditative state, and brain fog.

**Lemon Balm (*Melissa officinalis*):** One way sadness sneaks in is through a sense of disconnection. A plant ally like Lemon Balm helps us feel reconnected to life and illuminates the pathways back to our relationships. Indications include social overwhelm, big life transitions, nervous stomach, and general agitation.

**Milky Oat (*Avena sativa*):** There is a growing body of knowledge about seasonal affective disorder (SAD), including the important link between Vitamin D and SAD as well as genetic dispositions. I've also observed a connection between chronic burnout (or a previous period of intense burnout that was never fully recovered from) and seasonal waves of sadness. Working with a nervine like Milky Oat can bring the reparative energy the nervous system needs to recover and, in turn, help with seasonal sadness. Indications include feeling directionless, oversaturated with emotion, information overload, and compassion fatigue.

**Mugwort (*Artemisia vulgaris*):** Sometimes exploring our dreamscape can help us feel more connected to our waking life, which is where a plant ally like Mugwort comes in. Mugwort is especially good at moving stagnant emotions, including those held in place by traumatic experiences (which is why it can be a good plant ally to support therapeutic sessions). Indications include a difficulty connecting to imagination, nightmares, poor circulation, and sluggish digestion.

# The Lunar Body:
# Herbs to Support the Menstrual Cycle

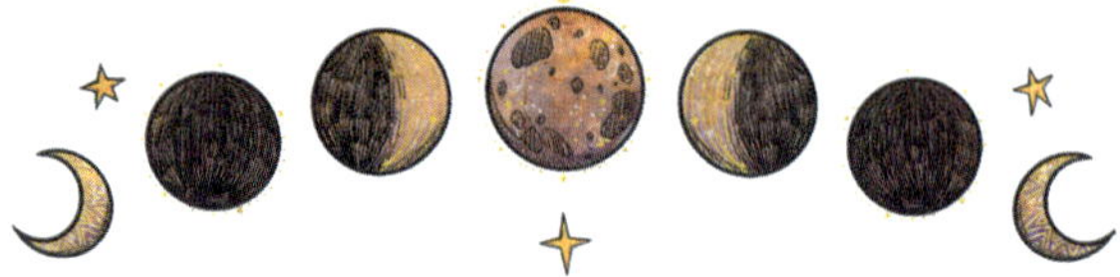

## *Herbal Actions*

*Hormonal and uterine tonics, analgesics, astringents, and emmenagogues*

A menstrual cycle that ebbs and flows with ease can alleviate a lot of the complaints arising when our hormones are imbalanced, from chronic pain to skin conditions to disruptive fluctuations of mood and feelings. While the following herbs are some of my favorite plants for general menstrual health, you should work one-on-one with a herbalist if you need more precise hormonal support.

**Cramp Bark (*Viburnum opulus*):** For those struggling with menstrual cramps, especially intense ones, taking a dropperful or two of Cramp Bark when cramping starts can stop them completely. Additional indications include menstrual symptoms that come on suddenly, anxiety, and general uterine congestion.

**Mugwort (*Artemisia vulgaris*):** A great overall menstrual tonic, Mugwort is useful for irregular periods, menorrhagia, amenorrhea, and premenstrual symptoms. Indications include anemia, nightmares, painful periods, insomnia, fatigue, fibroids, and cysts.

**Red Clover (*Trifolium pratense*):** Red Clover is a great first herb when trying to balance out your hormonal cycle. For menstruation, I recommend using it over several months during the week before and during menstruation. Indications include irregular cycles; hormonal acne,; canker sores; premenstrual symptoms, including fatigue, tension, and anxiety; and anemia.

**Shatavari (*Asparagus racemosus*):** Another great menstrual tonic, Shatavari alleviates common premenstrual symptoms as well as regulates menstruation so your cycle is not too long, too short, or too heavy. Indications include weakness, lack of energy, spasmodic pain, brain fog, and lowered immunity during menstruation.


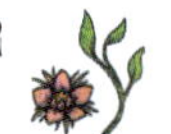

**Vitex (*Vitex agnus-castus*):** A menstrual tonic helpful in regulating menstrual cycles—if you have regular menstrual cycles but other symptoms brought on by menstruation, try another herb first—but if you have an irregular cycle, Vitex can be a great ally. Indications include uterine congestion, indigestion, breast pain, and hormonal headaches.

## The Midpoint of the Year: Herbs for Middle Age

### *Herbal Actions*

*Vitality tonics, immunomodulators, cell tonics, and anti-inflammatories*

By the time we reach middle age we've learned a few things, including about our body, what it does, and what it needs. There's still a lot of life to be lived, so we can turn to our plant allies to support our vitality in ways we may not have known we needed in our younger years. Herbs for middle age include hormonal tonics for testosterone and estrogen, musculoskeletal allies, and herbs that connect us to the dreams of our second half of life. The following can also be used either in plant form or as flower essence for healing your parental wounds or your inner middle-age archetype.

**Eleuthero (*Eleutherococcus senticosus*):** Eleuthero has a lovely ability to balance out essential bodily functions, from immunity to thyroid health to the nervous system. Indications include depletion of the immune system due to overwork, exhaustion from physical activity, hyperactivity, poor memory, and low stress tolerance.

**Ginkgo (*Ginkgo biloba*):** Ancient Ginkgo, with its brain-shaped leaves, is a great tonic for long-term cognitive function, improving cerebral circulation, memory, and vitality for the aging body. Indications include brain fog, poor memory, weakening sight and hearing, and fatigue.

**Mugwort (*Artemisia vulgaris*):** Sometimes in middle life what we need most is to reconnect with our dreams. Mugwort is a balancing tonic, helping all of our body systems work in harmony, but it is especially good for clearing out old visions and ideas from our dreamscape. Indications include insomnia, brain fog, restlessness, and irritability.

**Reishi (*Ganoderma lucidum*):** A prized vitality tonic, Reishi contributes to the overall health of the aging body. Reishi supports immunity; improves physical, emotional, and mental resilience; and enhances circulation, reducing the risk of blood clots and heart dysfunction while also improving oxygen levels in the blood. Indications include listlessness, insomnia, forgetfulness, dullness to the skin, joint and tendon weakness, hypertension, and general fatigue.

**Rose (*Rosa* spp.):** While I think that Rose is a beautiful ally for all stages of life, it seems particularly attuned to the challenges of middle age, when we know and have experienced so much but also have a greater sense of all we have yet to learn and experience. Rose is also great for the aging body and its growing needs for support for maintaining system functions, from effective digestion to restful sleep cycles. Indications include trouble connecting to current moments of joy, repressed anger coming to the surface, feeling disconnected from meaningful relationships, and feeling one's age but not yet being comfortable with that experience.

**Turmeric (*Curcuma longa*):** A great remedy to protect against the unwanted experiences that can come with aging from general debility, the growth of tumors and masses, and the weakening of the immune system. Indications include long recovery periods after physical exertion, joint and muscle pain, irritated digestion, and blood sugar issues.

**The Community Clinic in Autumn**

*Individually packaged cold-care teas for ease of use when people are feeling sick*

*Immunomodulating and immunostimulating tinctures to prevent or alleviate colds and flu*

*Warming, pain-relieving herbs mixed with Epsom salts for hand, foot, and body baths*

*Mood-boosting teas for those affected by the growing dark*

*Salves for arthritis and other conditions aggravated by the increased cold*

*Respiratory tonics for opening airways and clearing congestion*

*Herbal powder blends, like golden milk, for bringing in seasonal sweetness*



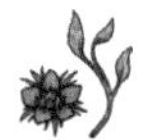

# *Autumn Recipes & Rituals*

## Energizing Autumn Tea

Support your transition into autumn with a tea that keeps you feeling grounded, centered, and focused. Herbs like nootropics, energizing nervines, and immunomodulators work to keep our energy up as the land draws energy in.

2 parts Thyme (*Thymus vulgaris*)
1 part Nettles (*Urtica dioica*)
½ part Ginkgo (*Ginkgo biloba*)

## Soothing Autumn Tea

After summer's levity, autumn's weather can feel heavy on the heart or too demanding of our time and energy. Herbs like nervines, heart tonics, and adaptogens help us to meet the season with grace and steadiness.

3 parts Holy Basil (*Ocimum tenuiflorum*)
2 parts Hawthorn Berry (*Crataegus monogyna*)
1 part Lemon Balm (*Melissa officinalis*)

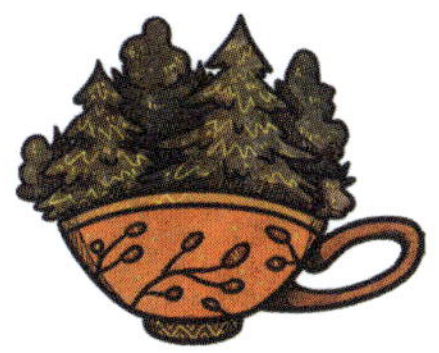

## Nourishing Autumn Tea

Autumn is a season of roots rich in vitamins and minerals that nourish our bodies through the dark half of the year. In addition to nutritive herbs, blood-building tonics and bitters help us create a nourishing autumn brew. The following blend is best prepared as a decoction.

4 parts Dandelion Root (*Taraxacum officinale*)
1 part Plantain (*Plantago* spp.)
½ part Cinnamon (*Cinnamomum* spp.)

## Harvest Blessing

One way we can slow down and settle into the interconnectedness of the land and all beings is through taking a moment to be grateful for and bless the people, places, and creatures making our herbal remedies, the food on our table, the clothes we wear, and all the items we use possible. I think the best sort of blessings are ones that expand our perception and draw us into action, supporting work environments that center dignity, respect for farmworkers, the greening of transportation, animal rights, and so on. While I've offered a simple harvest blessing with mealtime in mind, I encourage you to create your own harvest blessings that consider all the effort and pathways resources travel along, through both space and time, to get to you.

*Thanks to earth, source of sustenance*
*Thanks to sun, wind, and rains*
*Thanks to those who grow and gather*
*Thanks to all who travel the lanes*

*May your bellies always be full*
*May your medicines ever be sweet*
*May a life of hope and plenty*
*Be the place where we all meet*

*Blessed be*

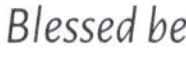

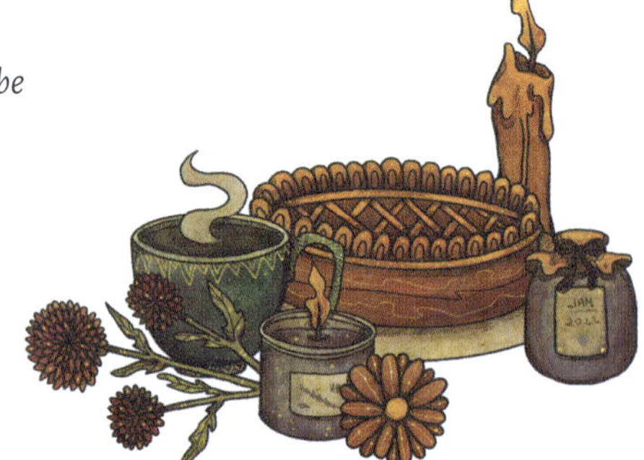



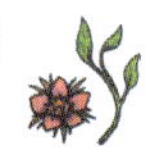

## Ingathering Community Ritual

Ingathering is one of the names for the autumn equinox, celebrated by many Pagans as a time of community joy. The following blessing can be performed during a community harvest gathering (though this can easily be adapted to any time of year or as an individual rite), and all you need is a basket to represent your community abundance.

Have everyone gather in a circle, and the first person starts with the basket in their hands, saying

> *This is the light*
> *The light that I braid*
> *I bring* [joy, stubbornness, laughter, food, etc.]
> *To this basket we've made!*

The community repeats the charm with the offered word. The basket is then passed to the next person and so on until everyone has spoken. Once the basket has been to everyone, it can be beautiful to seal the blessing by everyone laying hands on the basket together and/or directing the energy raised into the basket.

Throughout the year the basket can be brought to community meetings to draw energy needed for whatever task is at hand, and items can be placed in the basket (charms, amulets, items of clothing, herbal medicine, and so on) to gather up the beneficial energy of this Ingathering community blessing.

## The Witch's Oracle

Choose three plant allies, whether the actual herb or a symbol:

> one to represent your magickal self and deepest current of magickal energy
> one to represent your shadow self
> one to represent a place of growing enchantment

Prepare your space, making an autumn-inspired tea if you like, and lay out your oracle of belonging. Ground and center, speaking any divining charms you wish to. When ready, take up your herbs or objects, close your eyes, and either toss or place them at random on the oracle map. For autumn, I like to close my



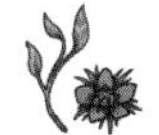

eyes and slowly spiral my hand above the oracle, in a widdershins motion, until I intuitively feel the spot where I should place my herb or object.

Where your magickal self lands represents the place within you that holds the deepest well of enchantment, intuitive ability, and skill at drawing dreams into the waking world. The place of the shadow self herb represents what we keep hidden from ourselves and others—a wounded part of our landscape we often try to protect with the energy of our magickal self. The place of growing enchantment represents some skill, path of learning, or philosophy that has sparked your interest and is somehow a bridge between your magickal and shadow self—though this connection might not be obvious at the moment.

Let's say that the plant ally of your magickal self shows up in the desert homelands of your oracle, representing how the strength of your ancestral lineage and cultural practices has nourished your intuition and sensitivity to energy. The shadow self herb lands on the place representing your lungs, pointing to a wound that may be connected to grief or your expressive self. Finally, the herb of growing enchantment may land at the riverways of your nervous system, signifying, in part, a recent interest in breathwork. The oracle speaks to a need for drawing from ancestral traditions to help you untangle some stuck energy around grief hampering your ability to express yourself and that spending time tending to the needs of your nervous system through exploring breathwork will support your healing work.

From the oracle you might work with plant allies with meaningful connections to your ancestral homeland, especially those having a special relationship to the lungs and nervous system. Choose one to three herbs to support your intuition, open up your energetic respiratory system, and soothe your nervous system.

## The Full Moon

Within the astrological roots of traditional western herbalism, the full moon is a time of cold and dry herbs, corresponding to the dryness of early autumn that begins to mingle with the cooler temperatures of late autumn. Autumn marks the harvest, the results of our actions, and the wisdom that comes with maturity. We can connect with this energy every month by working with the full moon.

In my own lunar practice, the full moon is an abundant time of remedy-making—especially flower, leaf, seed, and fruit–based remedies, as the full moon pulls energy upward and outward. I especially love making nervous system tonics, heart tonics, and magickal charms of all varieties under the light of the full moon.

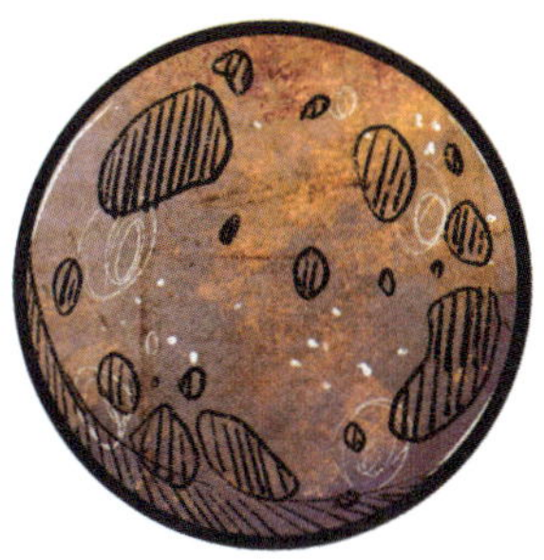

## *Full Moon Remedy Blessing*

To be said over remedies while making them, during their brewing process, or before administering them:

*By the light of the full moon*
*expansive and deep*
*cradle our healing*
*with energy sweet*

*as the moon dances freely*
*the remedy sings*
*bringing us hope*
*for all of our dreams*

*blessed be*

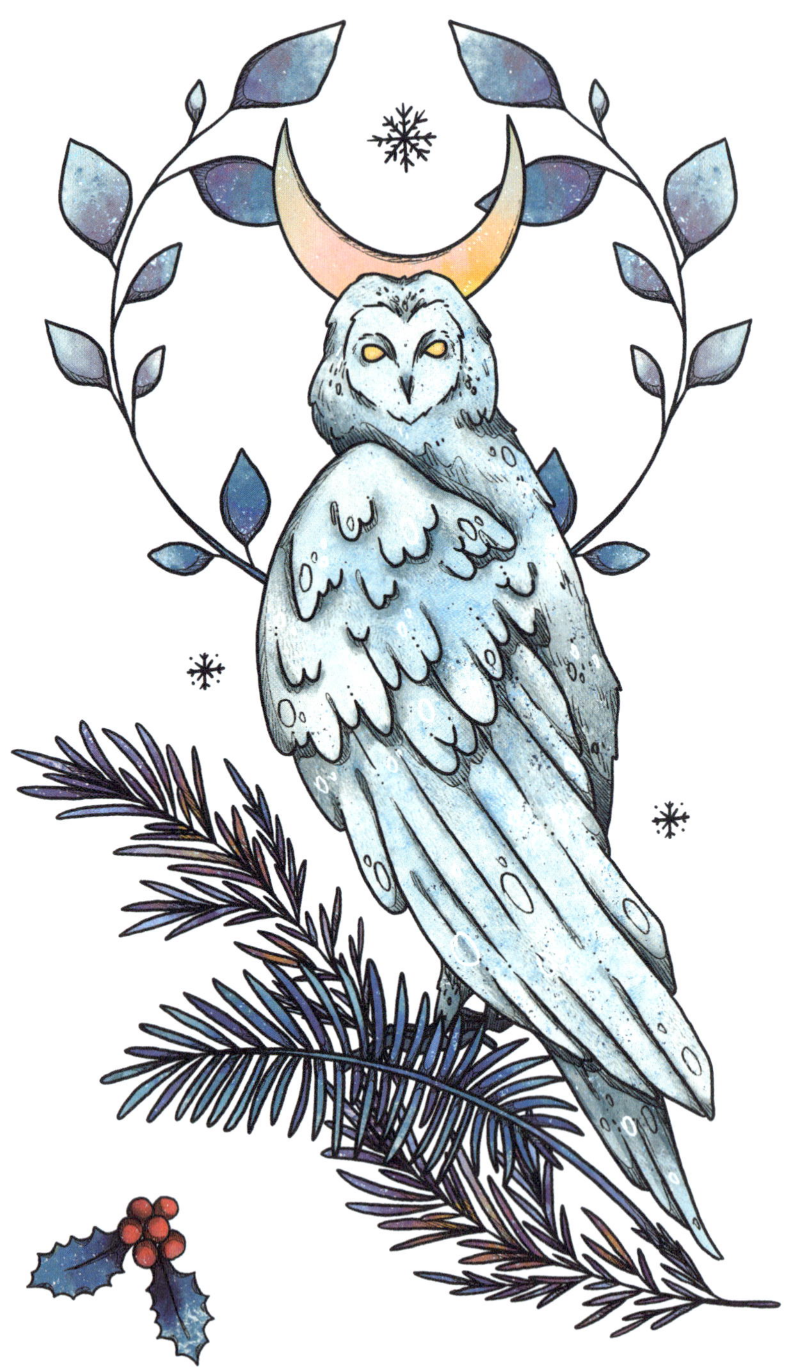

# Winter

Winter rolls onto the shores of autumn, the tide of light receding and the bare land coming to rest. Energy is drawn down into the earth, pulled by the season's cold and limited light, the sun resting farthest from its summer height. Winter is a time of gathering together in the warmth of each other's good company, remembering we are interdependent with all life and death on earth, preserving and sharing stories and food and blessing the bond between generations. The land is lit up by starlight and solace, in a state of renewal during this season of rest, tending to the seeds of future dreams and the deep roots of memory.

Winter is a season full of stories, and the dark half of the year is abundant with myths and festivities, from ancient reindeer deities bringing light and gifts, to fire festivals protecting against baneful spirits and variations of the sun being reborn through the effort of holy mothers. Winter lingers, settling around the boundaries of shelters made earlier in the year, slowing the pulse of the land to a resting beat so that life can regenerate below the surface. Coming to rest after the work of growth and harvest has passed, we care for our bodies during this time of increasing cold and dark by reaching for the steadying remedies of winter, from respiratory blends to immune system tonics and all variety of cold, cough, and flu remedies. The stories of traditional western herbalism tell us winter is when the energies of earth meet the energies of water, a period of fallowness and regeneration after a year of growth and harvest, bringing in a time of archetypal elderhood, the compass direction north, and the liminal magick of the waning quarter moon. As the energy of water increases, we flow into winter guided by reflected light, letting our feeling body find nourishment from the harvest of the past year, making sure to exchange that light with our communities so all are well-fed and allowing our body to move with the tides of our dreams and desires.

The decreasing light settles our energy, pulling us toward extended rest, and with this slower energy we need to take care of emotional steadiness, reassessing the legacy of our relationships, the ideas we are carrying with us as we age, and the structures that have stood firm or fallen with the changing nature of our life. Winter, depending on where you live, can be the quietest time of year in the apothecary, when the energy of the land is limited, the harvest done, and the opportunities for inner work and the exploration of life beneath soil and wave shine like so many stars and candles in the dark. As the land contracts and settles, our own energy pulls inward, and we have to guard against feeling separate from the dark instead of part of it and be mindful of the parts of our inner landscape most in need of restorative rest after a busy year. Opening our hearts to the land and our plant allies, our kinship helps ground us yet feels expansive. We look at what is flowing in and ebbing out of our life so that our healing work may be led by what we hold most sacred and what holds us in turn.

Where will our dreaming selves take us as autumn drifts into winter's beautiful dark?

**Cozy Autumn, Festive Winter Breathwork**

*Find a comfortable position, perhaps next to a fireplace, by candlelight, or even snug under a blanket. Let your breath settle into an easy rhythm. After a few rounds of breathing, begin to imagine soft starlight glittering all around you. As you breathe in, the starlight draws gently toward you. As you breathe out, it settles within your energetic field. Follow this pattern of gathering starlight for a few more rounds, then on the next inbreath feel your own inner glow draw up from deep within to meet and mingle with the starlight around you. When you sense a balance of light within and around you, feel your inner light pull inward to a comfortable place, glowing with the addition of winter's starlight.*

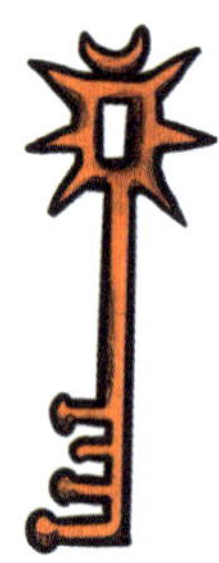

## The Gifts of Winter

### *Dreams*

In lands of deep winter, the year's growth slows on the surface, and even in temperate climates, the fecundity of spring, the rapid growth of summer, and the harvest season of autumn come to a pause. The long night of winter pulls us inward, where we can dream a bit between the end and the beginning of a new cycle of growth. The tenderness of spring is first conceived in the starry dark of midwinter, and dreams are the cradles sheltering all the possibilities of seasons to come. In winter we balance between our past harvests to support us and our future visions to inspire us. This is when the healing spell of dreams and dreaming carries us along, like ancient stones aligned with the solstice sun, marking the passage of time and our journey through space.

The farther you live from the equator, the more intense, dark, and cold winters can be—which is why you'll often find an abundance of therapeutic and community-strengthening myths and stories within these cultures. Through storytelling, the darkness is transformed from a tight, narrow space to an open stage of possibility. After autumn's busy harvest, when our maturity and knowledge have been tested and refined, the season's long nights are an opportunity to transmute that hard-won knowledge into the sort of wild wisdom born beside the warmth of a winter's fire. Winter is a time for exploring who we are and what we believe to be true about the world, as well as continuing to share, rework, or let go of the stories we were raised with. We live our lives not only shaped by our own tales, but by the reverberating myths of our ancestors and elders who dreamed of us long before we came into being.

The sturdy earth of our autumn bodies softens into the watery energy of our winter selves, and we can turn to herbs to support the fluids of our body, from kidney and liver tonics to protective and healing skin remedies. As in the summer, the winter solstice is one of the most common times of conception throughout the year, so fertility tonics are always welcome on the community apothecary shelf. In traditional western herbalism, winter is a time of earth meeting water, when the energy of the land retreats deep into a state of slow regeneration that makes possible all growth later on in the year. Through water, we explore the intelligence of our body's ocean tides, from physical to emotional to mental and beyond, experiencing the type of wisdom only gained through self-exploration and cultivating discernment in our relationships, letting ourselves ebb and flow throughout the land guided by our internal rhythms.

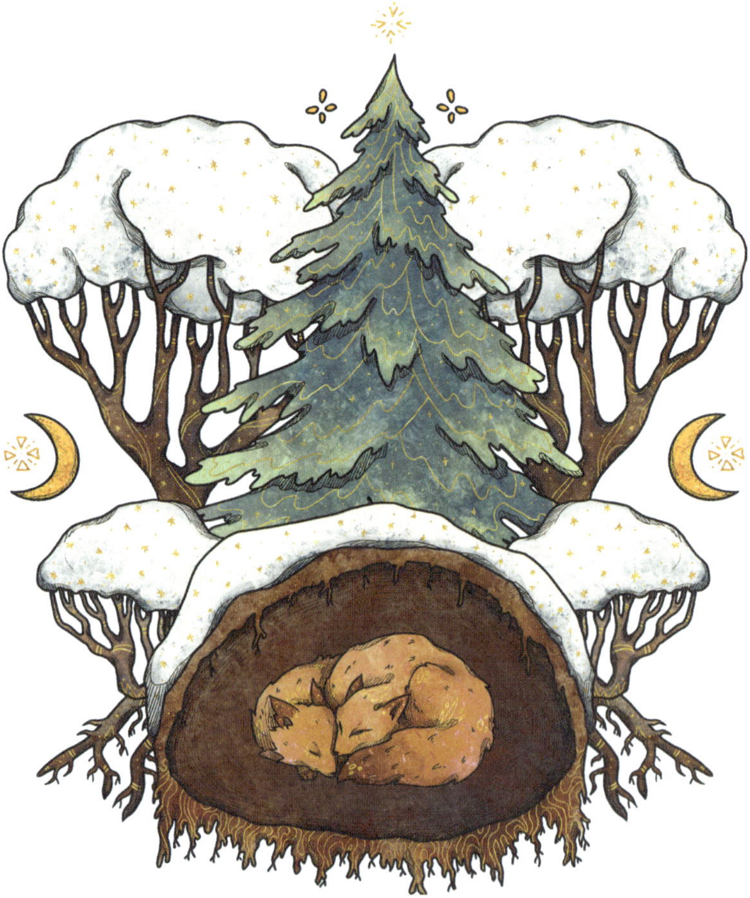

Winter's darkness invites us inside our homes, communities, inner worlds, and dreaming selves. The land is always dreaming: in spring vistas of new life, summer the bold visions of youth, and autumn the infinite among the finite. In

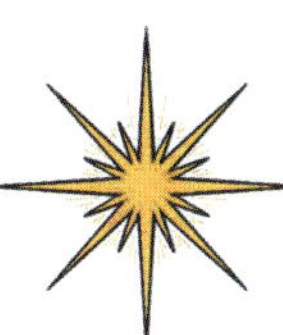

winter, with more opportunities to pause and be slow, we can take shelter in the land's dreaming, just like we sheltered in the summer's shade. Dreams also have a long tradition of use within healing work, with sleep temples serving as one early version of hospitals in parts of the ancient world.

I hold two intertwined beliefs about dreams. The first is they are personal physiological expressions of consciousness, generated by deep sleep cycles when our body attempts to process experiences and information, much as memories and made-up scenarios can appear before us in states of deep meditation or daydreaming. Yet I also believe dreams are not purely physiological, nor do they belong solely to the dreamer. A dreamer is a vessel whose dreams pass through. Of course, dreams are shaped by that passing and our unique form and perceptions, but they are also shaped and created by things far beyond our individual selves, from our waking experiences, the land we live with, our cultural references, and all of our relationships, from the stressful to the sublime. Dreams are one way we connect to healing's time-traveling qualities, when we journey among memory, present life, and future desires as we seek out well-being. Sometimes it is only through dreams that we experience a way of life only our descendants will live, knowing that the personal and collective healing we do today will help these dreams survive beyond us.

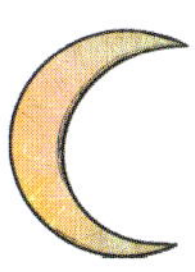

I love bringing the dreaming world into the waking world, exchanging dream stories at the breakfast table, in ritual circles, and, when appropriate, in consultations. Sometimes sharing dreams offers a gentler, nonlinear form of storytelling to name what is happening below the surface. Dreams are conversations between the inner and outer world, pulling us from the intensity of the now, with our illnesses and discomforts, to the healing wisdom and interesting possibilities lying somewhere before, behind, and within us. While dreams are not a diagnostic tool, they can be revealing, and I believe that dreams are one way the land and our plant kin speak to us. Even if we never talk explicitly about dreams in our consultation or classroom spaces, it's important to consider the ways we make room for people's dreaming selves to join us, much in the same way I make sure to welcome in a person's benevolent ancestors. In what ways are you making space for the dreams of those you serve?

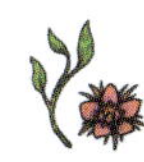

The long, cold days of winter are tenderly entwined with our seeking summer selves, but instead of going out to find support, we have an opportunity to draw in and become a sturdy pillar within our community. What we felt inspired by in spring, developed in summer, and tested in autumn can now become a resource to share around winter's festive table. Winter is less a season of proving or pursuing than a time of putting down roots and preserving our time, our wisdom, and our useful legacies for generations to come. The limitations of winter remind us that the land eventually ends and the sea appears. Guided by the energy of endlessly transmutable water, we can revel in knowing that after thousands of years existing with the land, the sea, and the sky of our planet, our species still has much to learn, observe, and understand in partnership with our plant allies and nonhuman kin. Through winter's wisdom we learn to discern what dreams to carry with us throughout the year, to guide us as we travel into known and unknown seasons of our life, and what skills and wisdom we have developed to pass on to others through our journey.

Physically, at the end of autumn and beginning of winter, it's common for our immune system to work extra hard as cooler weather draws us indoors where viruses are stabler and more easily exchanged. The remedies of winter are often immunomodulators and immunostimulants, general cold-care blends, comforting herbs cooked into nourishing food, and nootropics for clarity and mental health. As we dream of warmer months, we can clear out our apothecaries of old and expired remedies, returning them to the earth, as well as preserving what is left of the harvest in extracts (from alcohol and nonalcoholic extracts to liniments and herbal oils) we can use through next harvest season. Winter is also a time of working with what has already been made, from blending tinctures and flower essences to combining herbs dried earlier in the year into teas and taking general stock of what did and did not get used as we plan for the year to come.

### *Resilience*

The practice of naming, getting to know, and drawing our dreams down into the world is an interwoven process of developing, testing, and strengthening the weblines of our resilience. Resilience is defined in all sorts of ways, including less useful meanings that have become tangled up with concepts of productivity and morality, limiting it to a measurement of individual willpower and strength. Instead of a measurement of individual worth, our resilience is dependent on connection and community. We develop resilience through what is modeled to us, from loving relationships to challenging situations to building boundaries and more, and then we get to use what we've been shown, what we've intuited, and what we've never tried before throughout our life. Every season brings challenges, from little tests to monumental struggles, and we are developing our resilience throughout all of it, from little wins outside our comfort zone to experiences that feel incredible and exhilarating to the unavoidable hurt and heartbreak brought on by the ordinariness of life alongside systems of injustice. While personal strength is not absent from developing resilience, our ability to cultivate adaptable, sustainable, and healing resilience, to survive and then thrive after sudden or ongoing traumatic experiences by looking for and finding that we are being held by our communities and by the land—who know our wholeness—allows us to keep our sense of sacred self.

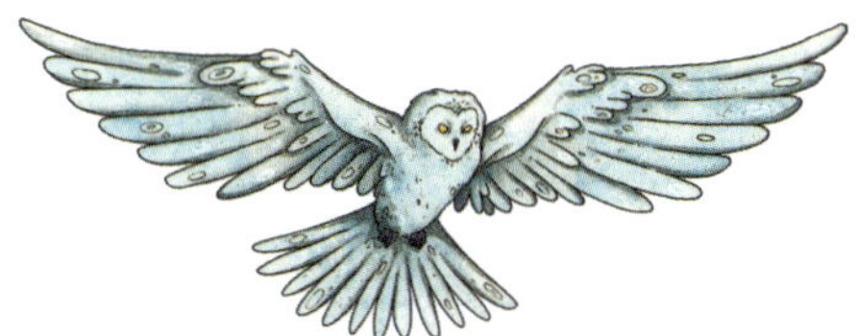

Winter's starkness—and increasingly any season's unpredictability in the age of climate emergency—reminds us of our fragility and the importance of a web of resilience to keep us steady and interconnected with our beloved community. In a practical sense, winter relies on the work of the rest of the year to keep our apothecary shelves stocked with remedies and the embers of our inner landscape well-fed. Winter also shows us where the gaps of our interpersonal and land-based ties are—when we have enough in the larder and where we feel uncertain about our ability to provide and be provided for. Lack of resilience is not weakness, but inflexibility—where we struggle to imagine what other options we have—and a rigidity that allows for little adaptation, leaving us frozen in place.

There was a point in my life when my commitment to the old definition of resilience, in all of its hyperindividuality and moralizing of health, fell apart. I couldn't hold it because it had never held me. I realized I needed to ask for and receive help. I had to unlearn a lot of what I'd been taught about how I was supposed to act resilient in relationships, at school, and at work. Being tough, not complaining, being the first one in and the last one out, grinning and bearing whatever challenge arose, along with not being "too sensitive" or burdening others with my needs, were all lessons I was told would demonstrate I was "resilient." Getting past many of those early lessons is something I continue to untangle, but the process has been helped by those who've modeled a different form of resilience.

Nowadays, I view resilience not as an act of eternal struggle against so-called weakness, but as a web holding us when we fall apart, lifting us up when we need a clearer view, steadying us in our uncertainty, and making it easier for us to do the same for our kindred. Resilience happens in the moments when we speak up about, ask for, give, and receive care and share our joys and accomplishments alongside our struggles. Resilience is letting ourselves belt out our song, trusting that we'll be heard, just as we are learning to listen and respond to the songs of land and kin. In other words, resilience is not the bell and how strong or loud or beautiful it is, but the sound made when it is struck. For those struggling to connect with the energy of gentleness and ease after years of overstretching yourself under the banner of what you had been told was resilience, consider working with plant allies like Motherwort (*Leonurus cardiaca*), Lemon Balm (*Melissa officinalis*), Rose (*Rosa* spp.), and Self-Heal (*Prunella vulgaris*) to start feeling into another way.

When we approach working with plants from an earth-centered kinship model, herbalism becomes a resilience practice. In my practice, part of modeling ways of resilience to my students, clients, and community is by showing gratitude for folks seeking help, asking questions, sharing knowledge, and settling into their vulnerability, all within a container of sacred boundaries. Gratitude is a lovely gateway to exploring places of resilience within a person's inner landscape and helping them not only find the places where they feel stable in their interconnectedness but also where they feel insecure, wounded, or doubtful of what


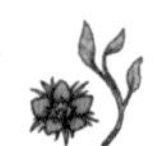

sort of support they are able to receive and give. Since herbalism really shines as preventative medicine, being able to recognize and name areas of personal and collective resilience is an important process of healing work, allowing resiliency to act like a social and emotional immune system instead of a measurement of narrowly defined goodness, strength, or worth. What are ways you shape your practice to strengthen your community web of resiliency?

The land in winter is the ocean beyond the gates of autumn's harvest festivals where life and death mingle together, where we celebrate cycles of rebirth with Midwinter's promise of light, but it's also a season of exploring the boundary lands of our grief. Grief is a common starting point for noticing our resilience for the first time as well as learning to develop the skills and connections resilience requires. Often we come to know what relationships, dreams, and practices are resilient in our life when we are on the other side of a challenging, shocking, or traumatic experience. Resilience can feel wonderfully present or starkly absent when we have experienced some sort of loss—around who we thought we were or what we imagined life to be to people, places, and beyond-human kin. How we are held or rejected through our recovery and grieving process is a reflection of our web of resiliency (and society at large), as a beneficial community response protects us and makes space for healing, while a harmful response from our peers often hinders us and deepens our wound.

While we can never quite know what sort of time we are living through, it feels to me that we are experiencing an era of collective grieving. We are living in a period of dynamic reassessment of the stories and systems we've been raised with, while also grappling with an existential climate emergency and the social and political upheavals that brings. Grief for the land, our communities, our bodies, and our descendants runs like a strong current through all healing work as we grapple with apocalypse. And yet, many of us have ancestors in the not-so-distant past (and for some of us in our very current present) who survived the apocalypse that colonization and imperialism brought, with its tools of war and cultural and environmental devastation, and that we continue to struggle against today. Our ancestors' tools of survival that many of us use today remain consistent: tight bonds of kinship with land and community, survival and revitalization of language, and celebration of life through humor, food, cultural celebrations, and rites of passage. While saying that we're experiencing an era of collective grief may sound doom and gloom at first, I believe it signals a vibrant spring after a long winter, but we need to live through winter first. Grief helps us map what was lost, what remains, and what can be dreamed anew, leading us to weave a tight and secure web of resilience.

When grief arises in my life, settling like an unwelcome guest in my lungs and heavy on my heart, and I am trying to find my way through its sharp haze, I am drawn to the edge of the vast ocean that lives within all of us. While many of us know how precious forests are for producing oxygen on our planet, it's the oceans and the life within them, from plankton to algae, that generate the majority of our oxygen. The lungs of our body are interconnected with the ocean lungs of our planet, so I am pulled to my inner ocean, my little sea, where I can look out over and under the waves to understand what I am drawing in, what is getting stuck, and what needs releasing as I process my grief so I can breathe deeply again.

Connecting with our ocean depths, the source of all life on our planet, is a way to meditate on our mortality—how short all of our lives are on this ancient rock we call home. Unexpressed grief, including the fear of aging and death, can devour our dreams, leaving us listless on the water, without sight of the land within or around us. Letting our grief move through us, our salt tears returning to salt waters, can be in itself an offering and a spell of reconnection, weaving us back into the web of life. I see resiliency as the outcome of an unhindered grieving process that has been allowed to flow freely, supported by the shorelines, riverbanks, and gentle harbors of community. Many lung and respiratory system herbs are also ones that aid in processing grief, and I often turn to plant allies like Hawthorn (*Crataegus monogyna*), Elecampane (*Inula helenium*), and Thyme (*Thymus vulgaris*) for assistance and nourishment.

These waterways all connect us to the predominant energy of water during the season of winter. Water is endlessly adaptable—flowing through our bodies, rising up in mountainous waves, falling from the sky, and bringing life wherever it flows. Within Western esoteric tradition, water is the element of the blood and fluids of our body, referring to our physical blood but also the genetic and energetic inheritance of our biological and cultural bloodlines. Working with



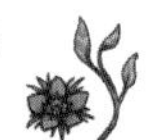

the water, the cradle of life on our plant, we develop an ability to resonate with the complexity of all life. In traditional western herbalism, the seat of water is the lungs, and water moves as Coldness, Stagnation (Moisture), and Relaxation in the body to sustain life. Herbs like Milky Oat (*Avena sativa*), Thyme (*Thymus vulgaris*), Passionflower (*Passiflora incarnata*), Mugwort (*Artemisia vulgaris*), Aloe (*Aloe barbadensis*), and White Willow (*Salix alba*) are all infused with strong water energy, supporting the water of our land-body.

Connecting with our lungs, including our breath, can be a powerful way to work with winter's pronounced water energy. Water is an element of emotional intelligence, empathy, and our ability to expand our perceptions and connect deeply with others—all essential for dreamwork and resiliency. When we are struggling to process water energy, we can find ourselves feeling brittle, oversaturated with emotions, exhausted, like we can't catch our breath. One of the best ways to support the water of our inner landscape is by letting ourselves ebb and flow with our energetic rhythms, taking time to dream, and protecting our web of kinship. Some of my favorite connecting and protecting activities include the following:

- Breathwork, especially combined with gentle movement
- Somatic forms of therapy, including dance, movement, art, and animal therapy
- All forms of water-based activities, including bathing, swimming, or aquatic physical therapy
- Making and using flower essences
- Any and all rituals of grief, including long-overdue memorials for people, places, and all our beyond-human kin
- Working with richly scented respiratory tonics that open airways, such as Peppermint (*Mentha piperita*), Sage (*Salvia officinalis*), and Thyme (*Thymus vulgaris*)

## Winter Inquiry

*What is my winter story?*

*What does winter feel, look, smell, and taste like in my body?*

*What does winter feel, look, smell, and taste like in the land around me?*

*When I go searching for them, where do I find my dreams within and around me?*

*What visions am I codreaming with my community?*

*What hidden dream am I ready to bring into the light?*

*How have I been shaped by the wisdom of benevolent elders?*

*Where is there unexpressed grief in my life?*

*What are the ways I am strengthened by and strengthen the web of resilience?*

## Herbs for the Winter Body

Within traditional western herbalism, winter is a time of falling temperatures and increasing moisture, moving from the dry coolness of autumn into the increasingly damp cold of the darkest part of the year. The land is slowing: Snowpack builds in the mountains, storing precious reserves of water that'll flow down throughout the warmer seasons, while the combination of coldness and damp draws the energy of plant life inward or underground. The moisture and frost of winter aid in the process of decay started in autumn, drawing energy farther down and inward, rebuilding the soil before another season of growth begins. Traditional western herbalism associates winter with the element of earth moving into primordial water, representing the final period of maturation and age within the human life cycle. Within our apothecaries we can support our winter bodies by incorporating immune system tonics into our daily brews, stocking our shelves with favorite cold-care remedies, including a variety for coughs ranging from dry to damp, brain tonics to support our seasonal mental health and agility, tonics to support our fluid-filtering organs, and remedies to meet the needs of our increasing age.



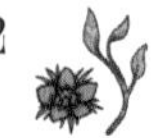

Winter helps us identify areas of our life that have become frozen, brittle, and lacking in vitality. Signs of Cold include weak circulation, ineffective digestion and absorption of nutrients, feeling understimulated, and an underperforming immune system so you're catching every cold that comes your way. Many recommendations for winter health within the herbal world and beyond include warming remedies from herb-enriched broths to hot teas to counteract the season's excessive Cold, which is why it is good to incorporate physically warming remedies into your winter rotation. When unresolved Tension or excess Relaxation from any previous season follows us into winter, it can mingle and get stuck with the season's increased Cold, leading to Stagnation. Stoking our digestive fires with warming bitters as well as including gently energizing nervines in our rotation of daily teas can keep us feeling relaxed but present. Slowing down and resting are part of winter's healing gifts, including moments of sadness and even somber introspection, but we want to guard against getting stuck in seasonal sadness or lingering burnout. Getting things off our chest energetically and physically (supported by lung tonics), sharing unexpressed grief, and working with plant allies as elders are all ways we can embrace and be embraced by winter.

Winter teaches us how to be watchful of muddy places that could become swampy and stagnant in our body, inhibiting the flow of energy. Signs of Stagnation include feelings of stuckness and malaise, buildup that results in conditions such as excess mucus or cystic acne, as well as general lethargy and even apathy. Most of us experience at least a bit of winter Stagnation. We also need to pay attention to the way we support the digestive warmth and fires of the body since the rich foods of winter combined with a slower digestive cycle from the long hours of night start to speed up again in spring. Signs of Stagnation such as bloating, constipation, gas, feeling like the food is just sitting in your stomach, and becoming overly tired after eating because digestion takes so much effort can be alleviated with digestive bitters and helpful energizing Tension in the form of astringent herbs that move energy. Late winter and early spring colds can lead to lingering congestion and an immune system needing extra support, so we can turn to anticatarrhal, anti-inflammatory, and immunomodulating herbs.

As a season associated with aging and elderhood, winter has us turn to plants with a special relationship to the aging process and longevity such as Sage (*Salvia officinalis*), Ginkgo (*Ginkgo biloba*), and Rosemary (*Salvia rosmarinus*). Through winter and connecting with the ancient energies of the land, we can explore the wisdom of our increasing age, learning to discern and carry only what brings us meaning and connection. Winter is a beautiful time to explore what inheritances have been passed down to you through the generations and the healing needs of your ancient self. You can work with the ebbing energy of the land, returning to the ocean lungs of our planet, by tending to your lungs, your own inner sea.

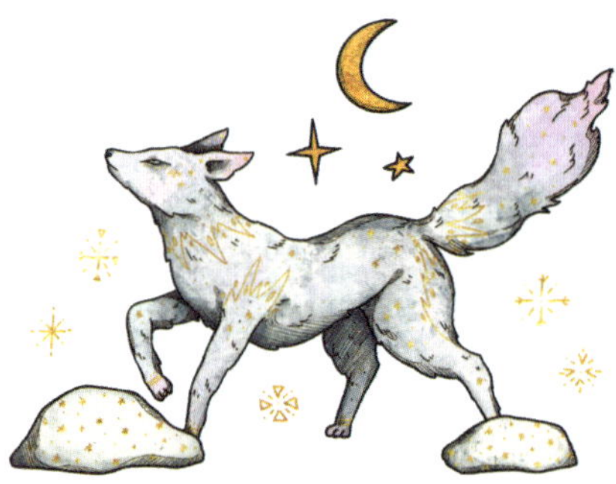

During winter, the land travels the path to dream and settles into a seasonal slumber. We can mirror the winter of the land in our own inner landscape, connecting with plants that support our sleep body, especially if our rest and sleep cycles have been disrupted during the busyness of the year. Herbs like Passionflower (*Passiflora incarnata*) not only settle us into a state of rest but pull into focus what really matters to us instead of what keeps us busy. Seeking connection with winter's rhythms helps us reconnect to our own inner visions, finding inspiration with the dreaming land.

# Winter Plant Allies

## Elder

*(Sambucus nigra)*

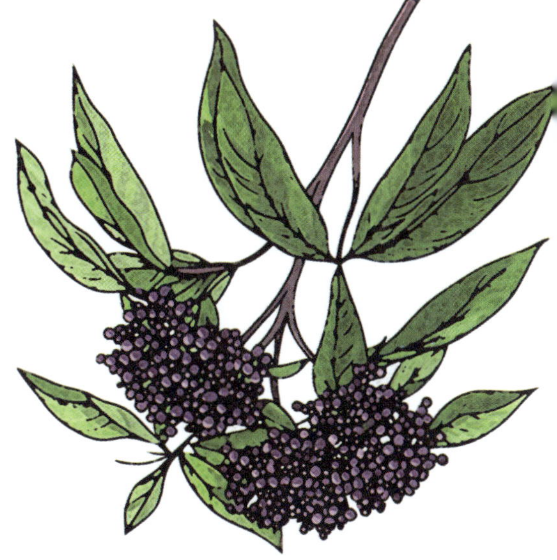

**Common + Folk Names:** Tree of Medicine, Old Lady, Old Girl, Hyldemoer (Danish for Elder Mother), pipetree, Lady Ellhorn, Fau Holle, Devil's eye, Danewort, fever tree, Queen of the Underworld, Saúco, Crone Tree

**Elements:** All elements

**Zodiac Signs:** Embodies the energy of Taurus. A remedy for Gemini.

**Planet:** Venus (in Crone form)

**Moon Phase:** All moon phases

**Parts Used:** Berries and flower. The bark and leaves have been traditionally used, but for many species of *Sambucus* (primarily the red-berried varieties) these are toxic along with the unripe berries. Elder leaves are still used within modern British herbalism in *topical* treatments.

**Habitat:** Native to Europe, Western Asia, and northern Africa

**Growing Conditions:** Well-drained loamy soil, regular watering

**Collection:** Collect the flowers in spring and the ripe berries in fall.

**Flavor:** Bitter, sweet

**Temperature:** Cool

**Moisture:** Dry

**Tissue States:** Heat, Relaxation, Stagnation, Tension, Cold

**Actions:** *Flowers:* Astringent, alterative, anticatarrhal, anti-inflammatory, antispasmodic, antiseptic, bronchodilator, carminative, decongestant, depurative, diaphoretic, digestive, diuretic, emollient, expectorant, febrifuge, galactagogue, immunomodulating, nervine, restorative, relaxant, vasodilator, vulnerary. *Berries:* Alterative, astringent, expectorant, anticatarrhal, antirheumatic, antiseptic, anti-inflammatory, antimicrobial, antiviral, antioxidant, decongestant, depurative, diaphoretic, digestive, diuretic, laxative, immunomodulating, nervine, restorative.

**Contraindications:** Generally regarded as safe

**Dosage:** Standard dosage

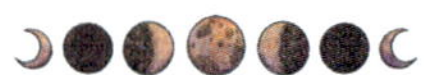

Known as the "Tree of Medicine," Elder has been cultivated since the Stone Age. Elder is the immune system herb I turn to the most because it can be taken over an extended period of time, acting intelligently in the body to disrupt viruses.

Elder is immunomodulating—stimulating an underperforming immune system or contracting an overactive one. One reason Elder is such an effective protective herb against the flu and other viruses is its flavonoids, which "bind and disarm hemagglutinins, tiny viral spikes covered with the enzyme neuraminidase, which allows the virus to penetrate cellular membranes."[22] Most colds and flus are helped by Elder, but primary indications include signs of fever, runny nose, excess mucus, aches and pains. The anthocyanidins-rich Elderberries also protect against and relieve UTIs and similar infections. Elderberries protect against oxidative stress and can be used over a long period of time to restore a body to balance and health.

Elder is a helpful circulatory tonic, pushing energy throughout the body. Elder opens and clears stagnation, moves the blood, and improves eliminatory function through the colon, kidneys, and skin. Edema, water retention, swelling, weeping and dry eczema, sprains with bluishness, difficulty breathing at night (fluid settling in the chest or constriction), and poor immunity, especially in winter, are all signs Elder may be useful. As a nervine, Elder clears brain fog and soothes the tubular pathways of the nervous system, calming hyperactivity and irritation as well as franticness and restlessness. Elderberries are also blood-building (helpful in cases of anemia) and alleviate stagnant blood conditions, helping to warm and move blood effectively.

The flowers relieve congestion, break up catarrh, and reduce inflammation. Elderflowers are also useful for upper respiratory complaints, including coughs (especially spasmodic ones), sore throats, tonsillitis, and fevers. Both Elderflower and Elderberry can be used to relieve asthma. The hot tea brings on sweating and can help break a fever, while the cold tea is more diuretic, promoting urination, alleviating fluid retention, as well as relieving night sweats and hot flashes. Use Elderflower for ear congestion, earaches, and infection. For kids with chronic ear infections and respiratory congestion consider Elderberry and Elderflower internally alongside Elderflower baths.

As a digestive remedy, Elder soothes spasms and cramps, cools inflammation, alleviates bloating, and clears congestion. Indications that Elder may be a helpful digestive tonic include signs of colic, heartburn, lower back pain, and mottled skin. Elder can be used as a uterine tonic when congestion and inflammation are present—look for signs of clotting and coagulation of menstrual or postpartum blood, cramps, and excess flow of thin blood. Make cool preparations of the berry and flower before periods for those who tend to overheat when menstruating. Elder can also be used in cases of postpartum hemorrhage.

Elder is helpful, both internally (berry and flowers) and externally (flowers), for acne, eczema, and gout. Externally, the flowers can be employed in facial steams and washes to promote clear skin. Use an Elderflower wash to relieve sunburns and repair the skin. Use as a gargle for sore throats and mouth ulcers. As an eyewash, Elderflowers can relieve sore eyes and conjunctivitis. As an oil, salve, or liniment, Elderflower is healing to bruises, burns, sprains, swollen joints, hemorrhoids, herpes, and hives. Use a cool flower compress to relieve headaches. The bruised leaves can be rubbed on the body as an insect repellent; test a small patch of skin first as some folks can have an allergic reaction.

### Seasonal Uses

I love using Elderflower in the spring to clear out congestion from the chest upward. The summer finds soothing teas made with Elderflowers and harvesting of the flowers for remedies for the rest of the year. In autumn, I begin to add Elderberry syrup in daily rotation to prevent cold and flu. Elderberry and Elderflower are always on hand during winter to add to cold-care blends, herbal baths, and skin-nourishing rinses.

### Magickal Uses

One prevalent myth of Elder is how it is unlucky and offensive to cut down or burn an Elder tree without the explicit permission of the Elder Mother, indicating the holiness of the Elder tree and how they should be approached with respect. Traditionally used to find witch folk, include Elder in charms and rituals to connect with the magickal community. Sitting beneath an Elder tree on Midsummer Eve may grant you the opportunity to see the Good Folk parading by on their way to their summer festivities. The Elder is a gateway to the otherworld and underworld; leave offerings to the Good Folk and ancestors beneath its branches. In general, Elder can be used in rituals and charms for protection, exorcism, and luck; to make wands; and to work with the Good Folk, ancestors, and underworld deities.

### The Elder Personality

Those who would most benefit from knowing Elder are often the ones carrying the greatest fear when it comes to getting grounded and centered in their life. Elder folk may appear to invite chaos and drama into their lives and make choices lacking in common sense, suggesting they may not have a strong sense of self. Those who love Elder folk often advise them to reconsider decisions that seem reckless or made on a whim without thought to their real needs and desires. There is a hollowness shaped by low self-esteem that Elder folk fear they'll find if they look within, so they seek to fill it up with snap decisions and chasing quick mood elevators. Working with the protective, fierce, and no-nonsense energy of Elder can help them recognize the importance of knowing themselves and what it is they really want in their life and relationships. Working to focus energy and connect with true desires helps Elder folk rebuild their self-esteem, discover


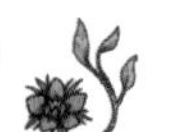

resilient forms of bravery, and learn how to relate in a supportive and constructive instead of destructive way. Elder folk are almost always drawn back into a grounded relationship with the land as part of their healing, coming through and back to community, carrying the spirit of the land deep in their bones, no longer afraid of being hollow, but full of song and purpose.

## Thyme

*(Thymus vulgaris)*

**Common + Folk Names:** Common thyme, garden thyme

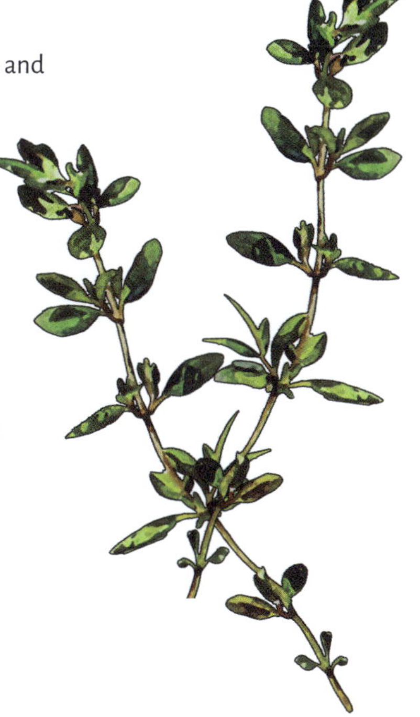

**Elements:** Fire, water

**Zodiac Signs:** Embodies the energy of Taurus and Virgo. A remedy for Capricorn.

**Planets:** Mars, Venus

**Moon Phase:** Waxing quarter moon

**Parts Used:** Aboveground plant

**Habitat:** Native to Europe, Asia, and North Africa, but widely naturalized

**Growing Conditions:** Full sun in well-drained soil on the drier side

**Collection:** Collect early in spring before flowering.

**Flavor:** Pungent

**Temperature:** Warm

**Moisture:** Dry

**Tissue States:** Stagnation, Relaxation, Cold

**Actions:** Anthelmintic, antibiotic, antifungal, antimicrobial, antiseptic, antispasmodic, antitussive, aromatic, astringent, bronchodilator, carminative, decongestant, diaphoretic, diuretic, emmenagogue, expectorant, immunostimulant, rejuvenative, rubefacient, sedative (in small amounts), stimulant (in large amounts), vermifuge, vulnerary

**Contraindications:** Generally regarded as safe, but avoid large amounts during pregnancy.

**Dosage:** Standard dosage

Thyme is one of my favorite kitchen garden remedies. It was purported to be one of the four ingredients in the infamous Four Thieves Vinegar, said to have protected thieves from getting the plague when they were robbing the houses of the deceased during the Black Death.[23]

Thyme strengthens the immune system without overstimulating and protects against bacteria and microbes. It shows up in a lot of cold and flu blends, especially ones to alleviate fever, because of its immunostimulating nature but also because it opens up the airways, relieves inflammation, improves circulation, and reduces fevers as a diaphoretic (i.e., it induces sweating to help cool the body). It is helpful with dry and hacking coughs, sore throats, general congestion, and asthma. I add Thyme to most of my respiratory tonics because it tastes good, is a great decongestant and expectorant, and clears out respiratory infections.

While Thyme is not traditionally categorized as a nervine, it acts like one, relieving tension and mental exhaustion. The herb also alleviates headaches and improves memory, cognitive function, and concentration. I include Thyme in many of my breathwork blends and love what herbalist Karen M. Rose has to say about Thyme and the breath:

> *It helps us develop a better relationship with time, connects us to our breath, and keeps us in the present. It is excellent for the fear associated with the out-breath release, causing tension and spasms in the lungs.*[24]

In other words, Thyme helps us settle into our practice while gathering our inner resources and loosening our worry that there is not enough time for everything needing to be done.

Thyme is also good for digestion; look for signs of cold and sluggish digestion alongside poor absorption of nutrients. Thyme is useful for times when you've accidentally eaten something you have a food sensitivity to (*not* serious allergic reactions like anaphylactic shock) or if you are starting to adjust your diet after identifying allergens. It supports the work of our filtering organs, clearing kidney and urinary stones, as well as assisting with overall liver function.

Use Thyme topically for skin conditions like athlete's foot, ringworm, *candida*, and dandruff. It makes a great bathing and steam herb as well as skin and scalp wash. Use topically for insect bites and wounds and as a compress or in a salve to open up airways. Thyme makes a great herbal oil for sore muscles and aching joints and an excellent bath tea for restless, overstimulated, and/or sick children struggling to sleep.

**Seasonal Uses**

Thyme is wonderful during the transition from winter into spring for clearing out lingering illnesses and opening airways. In summer, Thyme is especially useful for tending to the needs of the nervous system, helping to protect against burnout, and it is a great addition to wound and bugbite salves. I add Thyme to my tea rotation starting in autumn to strengthen the immune system and protect against viral and bacterial infections. Throughout winter include Thyme in your daily tonics to clear airways, help with colds and fevers, and support digestion with its gentle warmth.

**Magickal Uses**

Thyme is mentioned in both magickal and medical texts as an herb protecting against and relieving nightmares. Thyme also has long use as a ritual cleansing herb and is a good offering to holy ones, easily added to healing spells of all sorts. It's traditionally associated with courage and can be used in spells to increase the bravery of the practitioner. Herbalist Karen Rose mentions an association with the Sacred Dead.[25] Use in funerary rites and to aid the grieving process. Thyme is a plant of the Good Folk and can be cultivated in the garden to call them in and honor their presence. A traditional recommendation to see the Good Folk describes placing the morning dew found on Thyme on your eyelids and then lying on a hill.

### The Thyme Personality

I've often found two signatures of Thyme folk: The first is carrying tension so tightly it affects their ability to breathe deeply, and the other is being described as fae or otherworldly repeatedly throughout their life. Thyme folk occupy a space between the worlds more comfortably than most, can easily drift off into daydream (often as a coping mechanism), and see things from what others consider to be odd angles. They have often been belittled and bullied for their perceived oddness and can sometimes even feel like they're not quite human. Some readers are thinking right now, *Sounds like you're describing someone who is neurodivergent,* and you're not wrong: Thyme is a good ally for many neurodivergent folk. The Thyme mind can seem out of step with mainstream culture, and sometimes they try to protect themselves by denying their differentness or falling so deep into it they struggle to connect with others.

As an ally, Thyme helps folk settle in the present moment creating useful anchors to this world so that they can more easily move between their inner world and the outer world. The movement of Thyme is one of fluidity, adaptability, and respect for the individual's experience. Thyme helps them recognize their magick for the precious thing it is and learn how to breathe deeply into it, reassuring their nervous system, their heart, and their self-perception that their difference is a gift.

# Peppermint

*(Mentha piperita)*

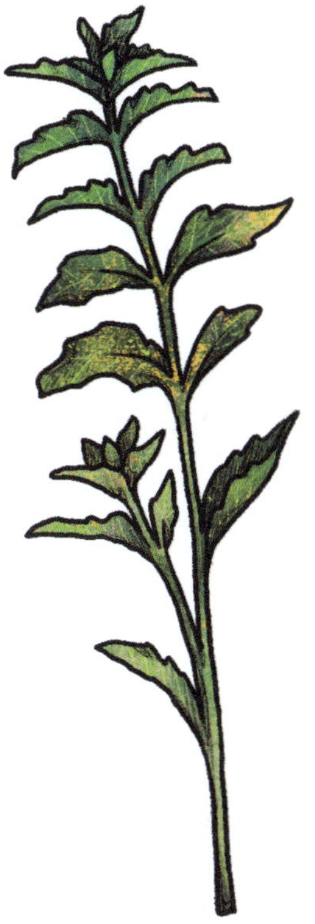

**Common + Folk Names:** Brandy mint, lament, water mint, wild mint, horse mint

**Elements:** Fire, water, air

**Zodiac Signs:** Embodies the energy of Gemini, Libra, and Aquarius. A remedy for Virgo.

**Planets:** Mercury, Venus, Jupiter

**Moon Phase:** Full moon

**Parts Used:** Aerial parts

**Habitat:** Naturalized throughout the world

**Growing Conditions:** Full to partial sun with moderate to high amounts of water

**Collection:** Gather in spring before flowering, but it can be collected throughout summer.

**Flavor:** Pungent + sweet

**Temperature:** Cool + warm

**Moisture:** Dry

**Tissue States:** Hot, Cold, Stagnation

**Actions:** Analgesic, anesthetic, anodyne, antibacterial, antiemetic, anti-inflammatory, antioxidant, antiparasitic, antiseptic, antispasmodic, antiviral, aromatic, carminative, cholagogue, choleretic, diaphoretic, digestive, diuretic, emmenagogue, expectorant, immunomodulating, nervine, stimulant, stomachic, tonic, vasodilator

**Contraindications:** Avoid large amounts during nursing as mints may dry up the milk supply. High quantities of the tea or tincture may cause heartburn.

**Dosage:** Standard dosage

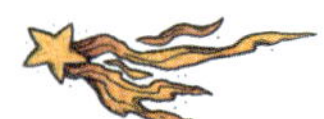

Peppermint is one of my favorite regulating and balancing herbs. A classic cold-care herb, Peppermint combines well with Yarrow (*Achillea millefolium*) and Elder (*Sambucus nigra*) for a symptom-alleviating brew. Since it is warming *and* cooling, it's effective for colds and flu with symptoms of fevers and chills. Peppermint strengthens the lymphatic-cleansing process and has been shown to be effective against a number of pathogens, including *streptococcus, staphylococcus, E. coli,* and *candida*. Peppermint's immunomodulating qualities are also tied to its improvement of the body's ability to digest and absorb nutrients.

The herb dries damp caused by excess Stagnation as well as expels mucus in cases of colds, flu, and sinus congestion. Peppermint is good for heart palpitations (especially when associated with indigestion, combine with *Crataegus monogyna*), inflammation and infection of the lungs, sinusitis and sinus headaches, asthma, bronchitis, and laryngitis. For bronchitis and asthma it is especially effective as a steam but can also be used as a hot tea to reduce spasms of the airways and clear excess mucus. As a circulatory tonic, Peppermint regulates energy throughout our bodies, releasing excess heat and damp, stimulating blood flow, energizing the lymphatic system, and alleviating brain fog.

Peppermint is a great-tasting digestive tonic and is especially effective for issues arising from stress and nervous conditions that lead to cramping, gas, indigestion, colic, IBS, and hiccups. Peppermint is useful for nausea caused by anything from car sickness to post–first trimester morning sickness. Additional indications for Peppermint as a digestive aid include headaches from digestive tension, lack of appetite, and distention. The herb assists with menstrual cramps and complaints due to uterine congestion. Look for a heavy feeling and bloating just before and during menstruation, along with mental fatigue and fog.



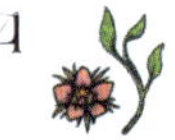

A wonderful nervine, Peppermint awakens the senses while reducing stress and moving energy as needed. If there is too much heat, Peppermint cools. If stagnation is a problem, Peppermint tones and stimulates. If overstimulation is present, Peppermint calms. I find it to be especially useful for brain fog as Peppermint entices and excites the senses to movement. Peppermint also assists with relieving anxiousness, nervous tension, and general anxiety.

Use a poultice on the stomach for pains and on the chest for respiratory colds. A topical poultice is useful for muscle pain, including back pain, and spasm as well as arthritis and sore joints since Peppermint is anesthetic. Cold compresses can be applied to the forehead for fever and headache as well as rashes and bugbites. A topical herbal oil alone or mixed with the essential oil can alleviate headaches when massaged into the brow. Use the tea as a gargle or spray for good breath and as a mouthwash. As an antiseptic, antiviral, and antifungal herb, Peppermint is useful for herpes simplex virus, athlete's foot, and other uncomfortable and infectious conditions.

### Seasonal Uses

For spring, I use Peppermint to clear out lingering brain fog. I love Peppermint in summer for its cooling qualities and use it both in internal and external remedies. In autumn I begin adding Peppermint to preventative remedies to protect against airborne viruses. Peppermint is one of my go-to herbs in winter as it makes most cold-care teas taste great and masks the flavors of more bitter herbs, making recovering from a cold that much more pleasant.

### Magickal Uses

Peppermint can be used in magickal works of prosperity, abundance, and good fortune, representing money and material abundance. Employ in rituals of cleansing and consecration as well as in incense blends to clear a space of harmful energy. The sharp scent helps awaken psychic senses. Use in spells and charms of clear communication, negotiation, and business deals while invoking the powers of Mercury. It is also excellent for magick concerning justice and the judicial process.

### The Peppermint Personality

There are two types of Peppermint personalities. The first tends toward a restless and nervous energy, with a busy mind and discomfort with silence. These types are able to chat with just about anyone, find themselves on social media for too many hours, and often tie their self-worth to positive attention received online or from outside of themselves. They have trouble settling down and being slow, and their anxious thoughts keep them up at night and restless during the day. What they want to accomplish every minute of every day feels dizzying and impossible. Working with Peppermint will help them get grounded and centered, learning how to connect with their stillness in a way seems true to their needs and experiences. Keen communicators, Peppermint will help these folks strengthen their ability to connect through story while developing a clearer sense of discernment for whose opinions and feedback really matter. When they are able to be fully embodied in their power, Peppermint folk are the type of people we need shaping our online spaces into better habitats of connectivity while also revitalizing the ways we connect in person.

The other type of Peppermint personality appears to be slow in energy, stuck in a rut, and uninspired with the state of their life and relationships. It is as if a heavy fog bank had rolled into their mind and they are unable to find their way to the shore. It's not uncommon for these folk to feel a real sense of grief for their lack of inspiration and confusion about who they really are and what they are supposed to do with themselves. Whereas the first type really wants to be noticed by their peers or strangers on the internet (even if they are afraid of what might be seen), the second type feels overwhelmed by the pressures of such perception and just wants a few close relationships (even if they are afraid they don't deserve closeness). Working with Peppermint can help these folks find clarity about who they are, the beautiful gifts they bring to relationships, and how to be seen in a way that feels sheltering and connecting. With practice these Peppermint folk bring the power of slow magick into fast places so that the process of connecting can unfold at a healing pace.


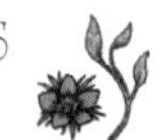

# The Winter Apothecary

## Clearing the Path: Herbs for Coughs & Congestion

### Herbal Actions

*Expectorant, anticatarrhal, mucilaginous, and sedating*

Life is carried on the breath, so it is good to have a few plants in our apothecary to open up the body's airways. Pay attention to the type of cough and congestion; some herbs are better at treating dry conditions and others more suited for damp congestion. Herbs for cough and congestion work well with nervines (see The Singing Land, page 70) and immune system tonics (see Strengthening Boundaries, page 201) to settle a person back into their breath.

**Elecampane (*Inula helenium*):** One of my favorite remedies for damp, irregular, and spasmodic coughs, Elecampane is an excellent expectorant and tonic for the lungs. Indications include congestion and excess catarrh, shortness of breath, sinusitis, whooping cough, hay fever, and laryngitis.

**Marshmallow (*Althea officinalis*):** One of my favorite herbs for dry conditions, including dry and hacking coughs. Indications include sharp and barking coughs, painful coughs, acid reflux, indigestion, and poor immunity.

**Mullein (*Verbascum thapsus*):** My favorite herb for dry, deep, and chesty coughs. Indications include bronchitis, asthma, general lung weakness, signs of adrenal stress (especially after long illness), and symptoms that worsen when lying down.

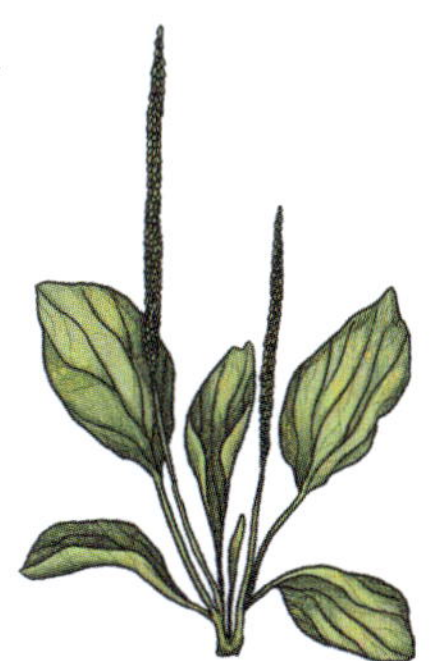

**Plantain (*Plantago major, P. lanceolata*):** A wonderful plant for coughs and congestion due to environmental pollution and fine particulate matter, including smoke from wildfires. Combine with additional cough herbs based on symptoms. Indications include symptoms that shift from congested to dried out, sore throat, and feeling like it's hard to take a deep breath without coughing.

**Thyme (*Thymus vulgaris*):** For coughs of all varieties, Thyme is an effective expectorant and immunostimulant. Indications include high and tight energy, asthma, general congestion, colds, and fevers.

**Vervain (*Verbena* spp.):** Vervain is a great nervine for excess tension exacerbating an existing cough. Indications include neck tension, headaches, hypersensitivity, and fatigue.

## A Sensory Feast:<br>Herbs for Ears, Eyes, Nose & Throat

### *Herbal Actions*

*Anti-inflammatories, antibacterials, antivirals, and analgesics*

We experience the land within and around us through our senses, so it is good to have at least one herb in our apothecary for every sensory system. Be sure to also reference Strengthening Boundaries (page 201) and Rain Is Coming (page 155) for herbal recommendations for pain relief, as well as the different seasonal allergy sections. Overall, Elderberry (*Sambucus nigra*) is a good herb to include in most remedies for the ears, eyes, nose, mouth, and throat.

#### Ears

**Dandelion (*Taraxacum officinale*):** Ear infections or inflammation often cause congestion and swelling, which is when Dandelion comes in. Indications include redness, swelling, and excess earwax.

**Chamomile (*Matricaria chamomilla*):** Great to drink to reduce pain, inflammation, and address infection, Chamomile tea can also be added to a bath, including foot and hand baths. Indications include signs of trapped heat, earache, restlessness, and headaches.

**Garlic (*Allium sativum*):** Garlic oil, typically mixed with Mullein (*Verbascum thapsus*), is a classic herbal remedy for ear infections. If the eardrum is not perforated,


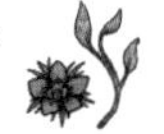

a few drops of the slightly warm oil in the ear can do wonders for earache and congestion.

### Eyes

**Eyebright (*Euphrasia officinalis*):** As the common name suggests, Eyebright, used internally and as a cool compress externally, is a tonic for the eyes, addressing issues like conjunctivitis, sties, and general irritation. Indications include redness and swelling, watery discharge, and itchiness.

**Ginkgo (*Ginkgo biloba*):** A good internal tonic to protect against degenerative eye disease. Indications include weak eyesight, allergies, poor circulation, and fatigue.

**Plantain (*Plantago major, P. lanceolata*):** Plantain is useful in removing fine debris from the body, including the eyes, as both an internal remedy and topical compress. Indications include exposure to environmental pollutants including smoke, redness, itchiness, and swelling.

### Nose

**Elecampane (*Inula helenium*):** One of my favorite expectorants for damp, congested conditions, including a stuffy nose. Indications include yellow mucus, respiratory infections, conditions that worsen at night and when lying down, and shortness of breath.

**Ginger (*Zingiber officinale*):** Warming and protective against bacterial infections and good for both runny and congested noses. A particularly good remedy if immunity seems sluggish and struggling to fight off a cold or fever. Indications include fever and chills, thin, watery mucus, and weak circulation.

**Peppermint (*Mentha piperita*):** The astringency of Peppermint dries up and clears out excess mucus and congestion all while being a very pleasant remedy to take. Indications include signs of excess heat, headaches, coughs of all kinds, and sore throats.

**Thyme (*Thymus vulgaris*):** A strengthening respiratory tonic and immunostimulant, Thyme is a great decongestant. Indications include dry and hacking coughs, sore throats, and congestion.

**Yerba Mansa (*Anemopsis californica*):** Yerba Mansa is a trophorestorative for the mucous membranes, making it a great choice for both runny and congested noses. Indications include spasmodic coughs, symptoms oscillating between congestion and runniness, and anxiousness.

### Mouth & Throat

*Note:* Many nose herbs are also useful throat herbs, such as Yerba Mansa (*Anemopsis californica*), Thyme (*Thymus vulgaris*), and Peppermint (*Mentha piperita*).

**Angelica (*Angelica archangelica*):** A warming and moistening remedy, Angelica is helpful for clearing out the underlying congestion and stagnation leading to symptoms like sore throats. Indications include general respiratory congestion, poor circulation, sore and raw throats, and conditions made worse with cold.

**Cleavers (*Galium aparine*):** Cleavers address inflamed lymph nodes and conditions like tonsillitis. Indications include swelling, hot and dry skin, lingering infections, fever, and fatigue.

**Lomatium (*Lomatium dissectum*):** My absolute favorite herb for sore throat and more serious strep throat. A low-dose herb only, take at the first sign of symptoms. Indications include viral and bacterial infections, respiratory weakness and congestion, chronic sore throat, and weakened immunity.

**Plantain (*Plantago major, P. lanceolata*):** A cooling remedy, Plantain works to balance moisture in the body, helping with both dry and congested throat conditions. Indications include lymphatic swelling, fever, respiratory infections, and general pain.

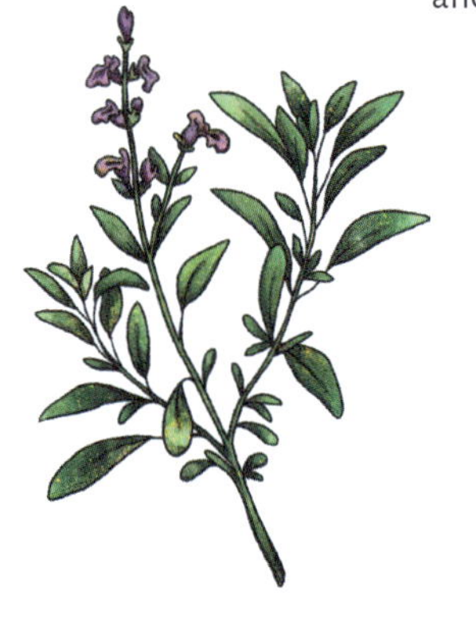

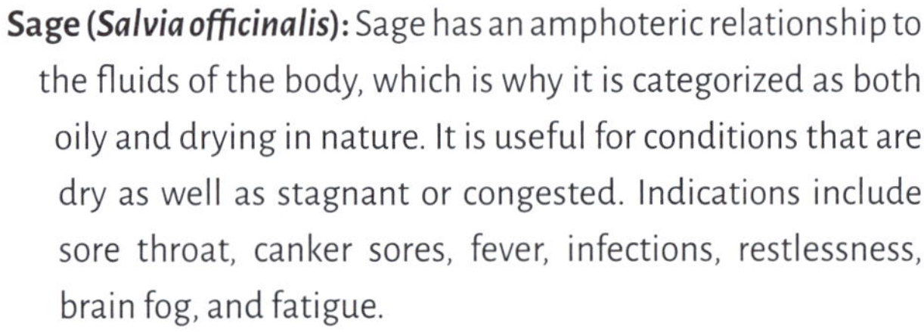

**Sage (*Salvia officinalis*):** Sage has an amphoteric relationship to the fluids of the body, which is why it is categorized as both oily and drying in nature. It is useful for conditions that are dry as well as stagnant or congested. Indications include sore throat, canker sores, fever, infections, restlessness, brain fog, and fatigue.

**Spilanthes (*Spilanthes oleracea*):** My favorite mouth and tooth tonic herb, Spilanthes has a wonderful way of alleviating most tooth problems. Take as a tincture and add a dropperful to water to use as a mouthwash. Indications include tooth and mouth pain, cavities, bacterial infections, and canker sores.

**Vervain (*Verbena* spp.):** A great remedy for reducing excess heat that has brought on swelling. Use internally as well as in a compress around the neck. Indications include ulcers, swelling, hot and sore throat, headaches, and general pain.

## Strengthening Boundaries: Herbs for the Immune System

### *Herbal Actions*

*Immunomodulators, immunostimulants, circulatory tonics, and nervines*

Learning the difference between immunomodulating and immunostimulating herbs is one way to become more successful at preventing and shortening illnesses. *Immunomodulating* herbs nourish and balance the immune system and can often be taken over an extended period of time, whereas *immunostimulating* herbs activate the immune system and should only be taken over a short span as prolonged use can lead to immune system fatigue. Immune system remedies are best supported by nervines, circulatory tonics, and plenty of rest. See also An Ounce of Prevention (page 159) for further suggestions.

**Calendula (*Calendula officinalis*):** Calendula protects against infection through stimulating white blood cells. It is one of my favorite remedies for feverish children and adults alike. Include in post-illness restorative blends, especially if the illness was long or someone is recovering from a chronic condition. Indications includes swollen lymph nodes, inflammation combined with damp stagnation, yellowness to the skin, and irritated skin conditions.

**Echinacea (*Echinacea purpurea*):** I don't use Echinacea often, but it is a powerful immunostimulant for short-term, acute infections. Begin taking at the first sign of illness, every few hours for the first few days, but no longer than a week. Indications include sore throat, fever, poor circulation, congestion, swollen glands, and repeated infections.



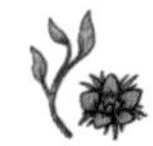

**Elder (*Sambucus nigra*):** Elder, especially the Elderberry, is my favorite immunomodulator. Elder disrupts a virus's ability to replicate while also strengthening the nervous system. I use Elderberry syrup as a daily tonic during the height of cold and flu season, but it is great in teas and tinctures, too. Indications include infections, fever, runny nose, excess mucus, and aches and pains.

**Self-Heal (*Prunella vulgaris*):** A great immunomodulating herb, Self-Heal appropriately enhances the body's immune response and moderates an overactive immune response. Indications include swollen lymph nodes, signs of trapped heat leading to swelling, low-grade fever, and painful joints.

## Breaking the Spell: Herbs for Fever & Achiness

### *Herbal Actions*

*Febrifuges, anti-inflammatories, analgesics, and immunomodulators*

Fevers help our bodies burn off infection, and as long as they stay within a safe range, herbal remedies can be a good response (typically, below 102°F for children and 103°F for adults). Herbs can also relieve the pain and discomfort often accompanying fevers. Be sure to check out Strengthening Boundaries (page 201) for additional support.

**Boneset (*Eupatorium perfoliatum*):** For times when a fever comes with "bonebreak" pain (i.e., intense bone-deep achiness), pain-relieving and immunostimulating Boneset is a great ally. In addition to tincture or tea, the herb can be used as a topical wash (especially helpful for young children). For best results, begin giving Boneset frequently at the earliest onset of symptoms, along with immunostimulants like Echinacea (*Echinacea purpurea*) to reduce symptoms and length of an influenza infection. Indications include congestion, weak coughs, aches and pain, autoimmune pain, and congestion.

**Elderflower (*Sambucus nigra*):** While Elderberry is one of my favorite immunomodulators and preventative measures for treatments against colds and fevers, I love incorporating Elderflower into blends for infections. Elderflower relieves


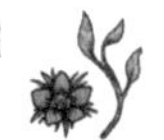

congestion, breaks up catarrh, and reduces inflammation. The hot tea brings on sweating and can help break a fever. The cold tea is more diuretic, promoting urination and alleviating fluid retention, as well as relieving night sweats and hot flashes. Indications include restlessness, irritability, insomnia, coughs (especially spasmodic ones), earache, and sore throat.

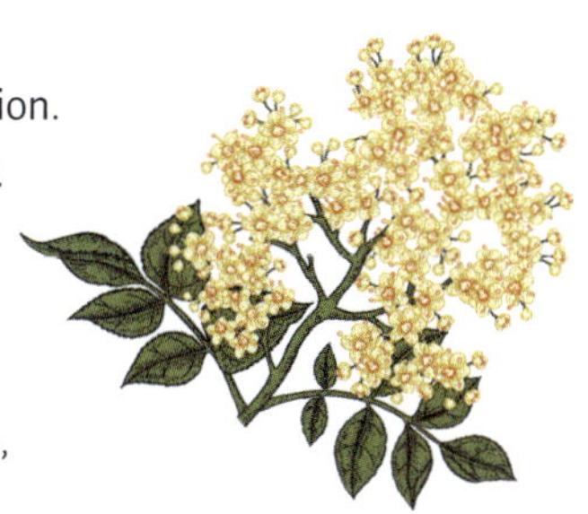

**Hyssop (*Hyssopus officinalis*):** A great herb for winter infections made worse by cold weather, Hyssop is a warming and drying antiviral circulatory tonic, addressing excess cold, tension, and dryness. Indications include excess mucus and unproductive coughs, cold and tightness in the chest, weakness in the extremities, and general melancholy.

**Peppermint (*Mentha piperita*):** Peppermint is a great-tasting addition to most cold-care teas and has the added benefit of opening up airways, reducing inflammation, and easing the general discomfort of being sick. Indications include sinus congestion, difficulty breathing, excess tension, headache, and indigestion.

**Yarrow (*Achillea millefolium*):** Yarrow releases trapped heat by improving circulation and opening up the skin, moving the body through a cycle of sweating, cleansing, and relaxing to reduce high, persistent fevers. Indications include red, splotchy skin, gas and diarrhea, rapid pulse, headache, and restlessness.

## Winter Winds & Deep Breaths: Herbs for Lung Health

### *Herbal Actions*

*Bronchodilators, antispasmodics, expectorants, anti-inflammatories, antitussives, and nervous system tonics*

The lungs hold the breath of life as well as emotions like grief and hope. Our ability to breathe deeply and move energy relies on the health of our lungs, and we can use herbs to relax tension, improve tone, and clear stagnation. Respiratory tonics and remedies are best combined with nervous system tonics (see The Singing Land, page 70).

**Cramp Bark (*Viburnum opulus*):** A great bronchodilator and antispasmodic that's not only useful for asthma but for coughs in general, Cramp Bark also has relaxing nervine qualities that address the stress and anxiety often accompanying respiratory constriction from coughs to asthma attacks. Indications include anxiety, cold and stagnant tension, muscle spasms, and heart palpitations.

**Hawthorn (*Crataegus monogyna*):** Hawthorn is a great daily tonic for folks with asthma, especially when accompanied by heart palpitations and triggered by general stress. It regulates heart rhythm and reduces stress as a nervous system tonic. Indications include general agitation, melancholy, indigestion, and people who are highly sensitive.

**Hyssop (*Hyssopus officinalis*):** An overall good ally for asthma and respiratory conditions aggravated by colder weather, Hyssop brings warmth and dryness to the often cold and moist conditions of the common cold, influenza, and other seasonal complaints. Indications include coldness in the chest, a general slowing of the senses, and weakness in the extremities.

**Peppermint (*Mentha piperita*):** A useful nervine and clearing remedy, Peppermint is especially beneficial for bronchitis and asthma as a steam but can also be employed as a hot tea to reduce spasms of the airways and clear excess mucus. Indications include signs of excess damp, inflammation and infection of the lungs, lack of respiratory tone, indigestion, colds and flu, weakened immunity, and dry skin.

**Rose (*Rosa* spp.):** When grief has carved a deep canyon, Rose can fill it with healing waters. Combined with herbs like Hawthorn (*Crataegus monogyna*), Rose helps us through the process of grief in a way that can feel open yet protected, opening up physical and energetic breathways. Indications include unresolved and old grief, fresh grief, general fatigue, anxiety, panic attacks, dizziness, excess worry, and feeling unloved.



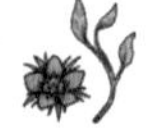

**Skullcap (*Scutellaria lateriflora*):** A beautiful nervous system tonic and antispasmodic, Skullcap is gentle enough to keep in your daily rotation throughout winter. Indications include overwork, nervous exhaustion, general hyperactivity, and lingering respiratory complaints after an initial infection (including the common cold) has passed.

## The Resting Body: Herbs for Sleep & Relaxation

### Herbal Actions

*Sedatives, soporifics, nervines, and adaptogens*

Creating a practice of rest and deep sleep is foundational to well-being. The roots of restlessness, exhaustion, and insomnia can range from the relatively simple to the complex, as our sleep cycles can be disrupted by illness, stress, structural racism, lifestyle changes, family obligations, adventure, and more. Here are recommendations for classic sedating herbs as well as nervous system tonics and adaptogens for more complex needs. With sedating herbs like Valerian (*Valeriana* spp.), Passionflower (*Passiflora incarnata*), and California Poppy (*Eschscholzia californica*), I recommend starting with small doses (10 drops up to three times daily) before trying a standard dosage.

**California Poppy (*Eschscholzia californica*):** If you're looking for an herb to reset disruptive sleep patterns but others like *Valeriana* spp. or *Passiflora incarnata* leave you too drowsy, California Poppy might be good to work with. California Poppy is less sedating but still relaxing, helping to draw energy downward. Indications include insomnia, tension headaches, bed-wetting, attention-deficit hyperactivity disorder (ADHD), and a dysregulated nervous system.

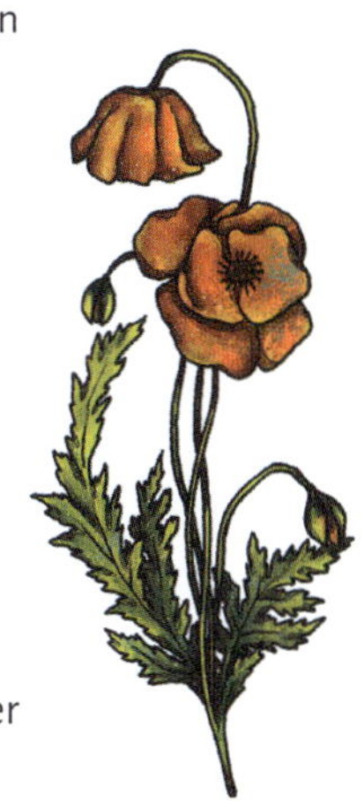

**Eleuthero (*Eleutherococcus senticosus*):** A favorite adaptogen to help return the body back to a state of rest. Eleuthero reduces stress, regulates the endocrine system, and strengthens our inner vitality. Indications include hypersensitivity, nervous exhaustion, PTSD, ADHD, adrenal stress, and recovering from intense physical exertion.

**Holy Basil (*Ocimum tenuiflorum*):** A preferred adaptogens to alleviate tension and anxiety contributing to restlessness and disrupting sleep cycles. Indications include excess stagnation, brain fog, weak circulation, and sore muscles.

**Lemon Balm (*Melissa officinalis*):** I love recommending Lemon Balm for finding that restful flow state during waking hours leading to easier periods of rest and sleep. Indications include tension, hypersensitivity, overextension of energy, stress, and postpartum.

**Passionflower (*Passiflora incarnata*):** A classic remedy for overworkers, the overworked, and those with difficulty taking a genuine break or rest without feeling anxiety or panic. Passionflower is excellent for insomnia, bringing in restful sleep, and helping you wake up refreshed. Indications include insomnia, muscle spasms, tremors, hiccups, pain, inflammation, and feeling easily overheated at night.

**Skullcap (*Scutellaria lateriflora*):** A great nervous system tonic and rest aid for those who start to fall asleep but get woken up by anxious thoughts. Indications include anxiety, overthinking, nervous exhaustion, and neuralgia.

**Valerian (*Valeriana* spp.):** When Valerian is effective, it's great for calming the nervous system and bringing on sleep, especially when there are connected issues of anxiety. For a small percentage of folks, however, Valerian can bring agitation, so start slow and if Valerian isn't a fit, try *Eschscholzia californica*. Indications include insomnia, tension headaches, muscle spasms, PTSD, and ADHD.

# Supporting the Process: Herbs for the Liver, Kidneys & Bladder

## *Herbal Actions*

*Hepatoprotective, anti-inflammatory, emollient, analgesic, antiseptic*

Our body is in a constant state of processing, filtration, and transformation, and organ systems like the liver, kidneys, and bladder do incredible work to maintain our well-being. One of the emotional signs that filtering organs need support is an uptick of anger and irritation as well as the physical and emotional body of experiences increased congestion. Combine with circulatory tonics (see Vigor & Strength, page 118), digestive aids (see The Internal Fire , page 64), and appropriate allergy support.

**Dandelion (*Taraxacum officinale*):** Dandelion stimulates the production of bile in the gallbladder and liver, reduces inflammation, and aids with overall functionality of the filtration organs. The root is particularly useful for the gallbladder and liver, the leaves for the kidneys and bladder. Indications include anger and irritation, acne, eczema, gout, abscesses, varicosities, muscular rheumatism, warts, slow digestion, sluggish circulation, stagnant energy, painful menstruation and menopause, and water retention.

**Marshmallow (*Althea officinalis*):** An incredibly soothing and nourishing demulcent herb, Marshmallow moistens dried out and irritated tissue throughout the body, including the urinary tract. Indications include signs of excess heat and dryness, feelings of sharpness, overheated digestion, poor absorption of nutrients, and constipation.

**Milk Thistle (*Silybum marianum*):** A good reparative tonic for the liver, Milk Thistle strengthens the liver, especially after a period of illness, stress, chemical exposure, as well as drug and alcohol use. Indications include yellowishness to the skin, dry and hard stools, varicose veins, hemorrhoids, irregular appetite, and hepatic pain.

**Uva Ursi (*Arctostaphylos uva-ursi*):** Uva Ursi is antibacterial and antiseptic, and is a diuretic; it addresses common urinary tract conditions such as UTIs and urethritis, as well as bladder and kidney infections. Indications include inflammation and swelling, fluid retention, hot and heavy periods, hemorrhoids, and incontinence.

**Wood Betony (*Betonica officinalis*):** Wood Betony is useful for stimulating the gallbladder and liver, relieve pain and discomfort brought on by indigestion, and easing anxiety. Indications include pain and nervous tension, headaches, anxiety, indigestion, blood sugar issues, cramps, and insomnia.

**Yellow Dock (*Rumex crispus*):** Nutrient-rich Yellow Dock stimulates liver function, helps break up urinary stones (but should be avoided in cases of kidney stones), and works to clear out congestion. Indications include itchiness and inflammatory skin conditions, anemia, weak digestion, gas, lymphatic congestion, and canker sores.

## Metamorphosis: Herbs for Menopause

### *Herbal Actions*

*Endocrine tonics, phytoestrogenic, nutritive, and anti-inflammatory*

Menopause, especially perimenopause, can feel very similar to puberty with all of the hormonal and emotional fluctuations we experienced as teenagers appearing again in middle age. Supporting the changing hormonal system and the emotional body and making sure that we are incorporating nutritive plants and practices into our daily life can all assist with this time of upheaval, rebalancing, and powerful transformation. Combine with herbs for the nervous system (see The Singing Land, page 70).

**Angelica (*Angelica archangelica*):** A great overall menopause tonic that alleviates common discomforts, including hot flashes, pelvic congestion, irregular and painful periods, as well as fibroids. Indications include general weakness, depression, brain fog, palpitations, anemia, indigestion, and cramping in the gut.

**Motherwort (*Leonurus cardiaca*):** Motherwort is wonderful for those struggling with the transition of identities that can become more challenging with the



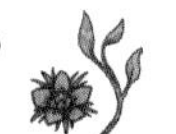

hormonal changes of menopause. Indications include stress, insomnia, emotional distress, hot flashes, low libido, and heart palpitations.

**Raspberry Leaf (*Rubus idaeus*):** A useful perimenopause herb to reduce the intensity of menstrual irregularities (including heavy bleeding). Indications include menorrhagia, uterine fibroids, cramping, nausea, and hemorrhoids.

**Red Clover (*Trifolium pratense*):** Red Clover is a useful phytoestrogenic ally for menopause, reducing uncomfortable symptoms like hot flashes, night sweats, and general irritability. It pairs well with Cramp Bark (*Viburnum opulus*) and Raspberry Leaf (*Rubus idaeus*) for cramps and perimenopause menstrual symptoms as well as Shatavari (*Asparagus racemosus*) for endocrine system support. Indications include hot and dry skin conditions, hormonal acne, constipation, and overall increased sensitivity.

**Rose (*Rosa* spp.):** During big life transitions turning to the wisdom of our plant ancestors can help us through whatever challenges we face. Rose is an ancient plant and wise ally for navigating menopause and its vast changes to our place in the world, relationships, and inner landscape. Indications include emotional tension, anxiety that creates tightness in the chest, fear of change, irregular menstruation, hot flashes, uterine spasm, and congestion.

**Sage (*Salvia officinalis*):** Not only does Sage help to welcome us into the wisdom of our second half of life, but it is a wonderful remedy for hot flashes and night sweats. Sage is a great aging tonic, strengthening our resilience for decades to come. Indications include fatigue, chronic infections, excess sweating, gas and indigestion, headaches, and depression.

**Skullcap (*Scutellaria lateriflora*):** Change is challenging at the best of times but can be especially hard when accompanied by intense bodily fluctuations. Skullcap is a loving ally for those who need help riding the wave of menopause with greater ease and empowerment. Indications include anxiety, fear, nervous tension, and the desire to do something brave with one's life.

# The Eldership of the Year: Herbs for Seniors

## *Herbal Actions*

*Nootropics, immunomodulators, and rejuvenatives*

Without elders there would be no plant wisdom, so working with plants in our senior years holds a special magick. Aging bodies have many needs, so be sure to check out specific sections of each season's apothecary to find more focused support for a body system. The herbs I recommend here are ones that help us feel connected to our vitality, support our longevity, and nourish cognition.

**Gotu Kola (*Centella asiatica*):** A good long-term brain tonic for cognition and alleviating fatigue, Gotu Kola improves memory, elevates mood, and increases mental adaptability. A really excellent ally for neurodiverse elders. Indications include senility, anxiety, depression, sluggish digestion, brain fog, adrenal stress, fibromyalgia, post-surgery recovery needs, and water retention.

**Holy Basil (*Ocimum tenuiflorum*):** I love Holy Basil as an adaptogen for seniors because it gently but effectively moves energy throughout the body, helping to address stagnation, clear brain fog, and support cognition. Indications include overstimulation, tension and anxiety, chronic coughs, asthma, and allergies.

**Milky Oat (*Avena sativa*):** A lifelong ally, Milky Oat shines as a restorative for the senior nervous system. It can take longer to recover from common or more serious illnesses as we age, placing extra stress on the nervous system; Milky Oat assists with that recovery and regeneration process. Indications include fatigue, melancholy, insomnia, overwork (including struggles with embracing retirement), and debilitation after illness.

**Rhodiola (*Rhodiola rosea*):** My favorite adaptogen and endocrine tonic for elders, Rhodiola is an excellent tonic for mental clarity, vitality, and energy. The herb also helps with healthy circulation, heart function, and physical energy. Indications include stress, burnout, fatigue, depression, poor memory and concentration, recovering from chemotherapy or radiation therapy, lowered immunity, and adrenal stress.



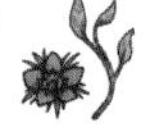

**Rose (*Rosa* spp.):** I like to work with plant elders when creating remedies for human elders, and Rose is a favorite herb to turn to. Rose is useful for all body systems but also supports the blossoming of our inner landscape, bringing joy and hope to places of deepest shadow. Indications include excess inflammation, autoimmune conditions, and fluid imbalances that lead to depletion of energy and blood in the body, including diarrhea, excess bleeding, and water retention.

**The Community Clinic in Winter**

*Cold-care packages that include febrifuge, cough, and decongestant blends*
*Herbal chest rubs and steams to clear respiratory congestion*
*Warming herbal body and foot baths to improve circulation and post-illness health*
*Spiced tea blends to improve immunity and lift mood*
*Digestive bitters that support our ability to process food and feelings*
*Blends for seasonal sadness and increased stress due to social and family gatherings*
*Herbal remedies, including lavender pillows, to assist with healthy sleep cycles*

# *Winter Recipes & Rituals*

## Energizing Winter Tea

Support your transition into winter with a tea that helps you feel focused, present, and able to participate in the season's cheer in an energetically sustainable way. Herbs like circulatory tonics, warming bitters, and nootropics keep our spirits up.

2 parts Peppermint (*Mentha piperita*)
1 part Rosemary (*Salvia rosmarinus*)
Fresh Ginger (*Zingiber officinale*) to taste

## Soothing Winter Tea

Sometimes winter feels too slow, too quiet, or like you can't quite find your rhythm of rest. Herbs like gentle sedatives, relaxing adaptogens, and uplifting heart tonics can help us feel part of winter's glow, instead of lost in the dark.

2 parts Holy Basil (*Ocimum tenuiflorum*)
½ part Rose (*Rosa* spp.)
Pinch of Cinnamon (*Cinnamomum* spp.) per serving

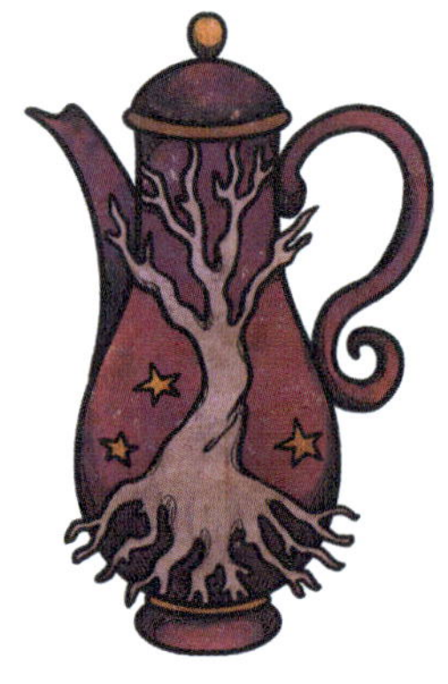

## Nourishing Winter Tea

Winter is a season full of the year's harvest, but nutrient-rich berries that protect us against illness and uplift our spirits during the long dark of the year can be particularly powerful. Vitamin-rich respiratory tonics and rejuvenative herbs are all welcome in a nourishing winter blend.

2 parts Elderberry (*Sambucus nigra*)
1 part Thyme (*Thymus vulgaris*)
½ part Hawthorn Berry (*Crataegus monogyna*)

## Land-Body Blessing

Body blessings are abundant in feminist traditions of witchcraft and spirituality because they are such a simple and powerful way to break hexes of self-loathing and plant seeds of body-possibility.

A Land-Body Blessing focuses on naming different parts of yourself with earth-centered language as a form of empowerment. While I've written an example blessing, I encourage you to write your own unique one that incorporates language reflecting the uniqueness of your form, the lands you feel kinship with, and words that are empowering and hex-shattering. The Land-Body Blessing can be used at any time, including before consulting your oracle of belonging or any rites of magick. The blessing can also be turned into a full ritual, complete with plant allies in the form of a sacred bath, anointing oil, body spray, tea, incense, and more.

*Blessed be the rivers of my blood*
*The deep sea of my womb*
*My rock-curved feet*
*My heart rose in bloom*

*Blessed be my stormy brows*
*the mountains of my shoulders*
*my honeysuckle vines of hair*
*my bones of quartz and boulder*

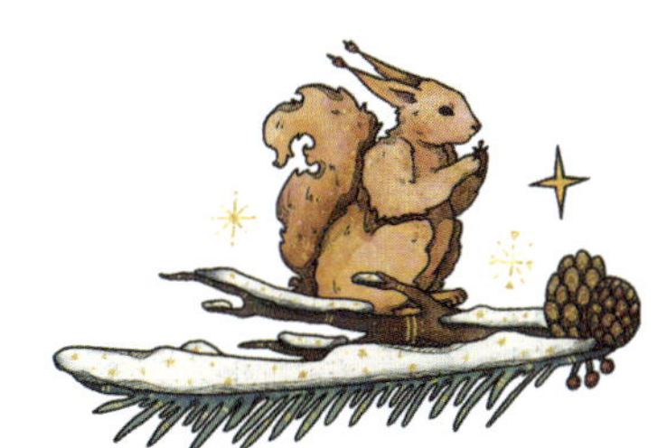

*Blessed be my crowsong voice*
*The wildflower hills of my thighs*
*My curving full moon belly*
*My lightning-flash eyes*

*Blessed be my forest lungs*
*The grasslands of my skin*
*My brain cell mycelium*
*My loud and thunderous grin*

*Blessed be all parts of me*
*my homeland*
*my land-body*

## Dead Stories Ritual

Winter straddles the waves between the lands of the living and the dead, creating an interesting atmosphere of liberation from the typical rhythms of the year, including from what we've brought with us into the dark. There are moments in life when we realize we're telling a story that has become dead—we continue because it is comfortable or convenient, we're fearful of what another story might mean, or any other reason we come up with to choose what was over what is becoming. The Dead Stories Ritual helps us bury these stories with honor, letting them decay so they may be fodder for future stories better reflecting who we know ourselves to be and how we want to be known by the land of our body and our beloved communities.

Dead Stories is a good ritual for before and during big transitions when grief and unease can arise as new and appropriate boundaries are being set in your life (e.g., getting out of an abusive relationship, starting therapy, self-acceptance, identity transitions, etc.). These are ultimately joyful moments, but often we need to honor our grief and fear through acknowledging and releasing these dead stories before we can access that joy. This is a great ritual to perform on your own or with your beloved community. It should be adapted to your needs,

and you should shape it in the way that makes the most sense to you—for these are your stories to bury and your stories to tell.

**You will need:**

Paper and pen
A metal cauldron or burn-safe container
Incense tongs
A bowl of water (moon water, spring water, water from melted snow, herb- or flower essence-infused water, etc.)
A washcloth
An herbal anointing oil of your choosing
A living stories altar with one or more candles (see description below.)

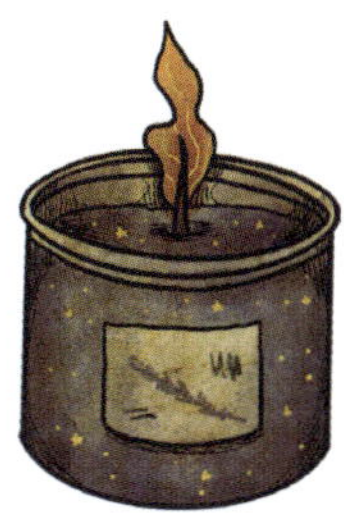

You will need two altar spaces: one in front of you and one behind you. The space in front of you is the dead stories altar and should hold your paper, pen, burn-safe container, and nothing more. The space behind you is where you can build your living stories altar filled with items representing what you are bringing into your life, including your herbal anointing oil. If you need help exploring any of these stories during the ritual, feel free to turn to your oracle of choice to guide you.

Begin by writing the old story down on your paper. Take as little or as long as you like—feeling this story as it is moving through your body, through the pen, and onto the page. I encourage you to do this in silence to represent the way this dead story has silenced other living stories in your life. When your story is written, begin to tear the paper into shreds, initiating the process of decay. This is when you can start to make sound if you're called to it—no words yet, but feeling-sounds and grieving-sounds.

Add the shredded dead story paper to your cauldron and light the pieces on fire. Use the tongs to make sure all the paper burns.

When the body of the dead story has turned to ash, representing its transformation into something new, and it is cool enough to touch, you can start to rub the ash against your forehead or any part of your body you choose. At this time you (or your community) can start to call forth the living story from within you, all with affirming language. Examples of solo and/or community phrasing include:

> *Hello, sweet soft little me, you're safe now.*
> *My name is* [name] *and I am* [brave, smart, wise, beautiful, etc.].
> *I am* [chosen name]. [Chosen name] *is my name.*
> [Chosen name] *is who I am.*
> *There you are! You're so brave! We've been waiting for you! Come on home!*
> *Oh we've been waiting for you,* [chosen name].
> *Come on home,* [name], *tell us your story. We've missed you!*

Once the ash has been rubbed on your forehead or elsewhere, pick up the washcloth and submerge it in the water. Use the cloth to wash the ash off of you. If you are in a community ritual and feel comfortable with it, have one or more members of the community wash the ash off for you. Wordless songs or comforting humming by you and/or your community can harmonize your living story in your body.

When you are ready, turn for the first time to your living story altar, pick up the oil and anoint your forehead where the ash was. From here you can speak and laugh and say what you please. Light the candles on your new story altar and speak your new story, new name, new career, new beliefs about yourself. You did it! It can be very sweet and grounding to have a feast of favorite foods prepared for after this rite. Any leftover ash should be buried, flushed, or disposed of in a way that feels final.

## The Ancestor's Oracle

Choose three plant allies, whether the actual herb or a symbol:

> one for your ancient self connected to your ancestors
> one for where you are holding fear
> one for a spark of hope

Prepare your space, making a winter-inspired tea if you like, and lay out your oracle of belonging before you. Ground and center, speaking any divining charms you wish to. When ready, take up your herbs or objects, close your eyes, and either toss or place them at random on the oracle map. For winter, I like to lay out my herbs or charms before me, soften my gaze, and then one by one ask my ancestor(s) to guide my hand to choose and place each herb or charm on the oracle.

Where the plant of your ancient self lands symbolizes either a genetic or energetic inheritance from your ancestors that is now showing up strongly in your healing practice. The place the herb of fear lands illuminates a body system that is most affected by this tension. Finally, the placement of the plant ally of hope points to an area of your life that can be supported in generating a greater sense of possibility for what might be.

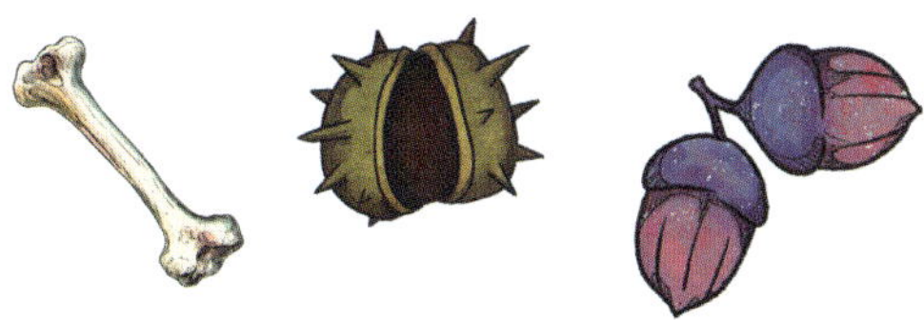

Let's say the plant ally of your ancient self lands in the place of bones, perhaps drawing your attention to your actual skeletal structure or more broadly to what you "feel in your bones" about who you are and where you come from. The herb of holding fear landing in the cave of memory might point to anxieties stirred up by intergenerational trauma or even your own early memories.

The herb of hope landing at the place on a hedgerow, representing both liminal spaces and ways you have learned to protect yourself and create boundaries, may point to spending more time conversing with your ancestors (e.g., a nightly ancestor practice) but also to the skills you already have to keep yourself whole and thriving and all the ways you've done just that.

From this oracle you might choose to work with plant allies of your ancestral line, if possible, but also consider herbs that help us process our experiences, such as nootropics and nervines. Consider choosing one to three herbs that are nutritive (a place of bones points to bone-building minerals and vitamins), alleviate anxiety, and help you feel deeply loved.

## The Waning Quarter Moon

Within the astrological roots of traditional western herbalism, the waning quarter moon is a time of cold and moist herbs, corresponding to the increasing cold and damp winter brings. Winter is a season of the dreaming land, when life on the surface slows, but our inner landscapes brighten with visions of what has been and what may come to pass. Each month the waning quarter moon carries this energy of dream and liminality, strengthening our ability to explore our inner worlds and the pathways of our community web with greater ease.

In my own lunar practice, I enjoy harvesting plants and making remedies that correspond to the energies of liminality, helping us care for the ways impermanence has marked and shaped us, including nootropic blends that turn the tide of forgetting and strengthen memory as well as nervous system tonics and more magickal blends to process the feelings that arise when we return from these liminal spaces.



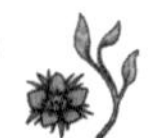

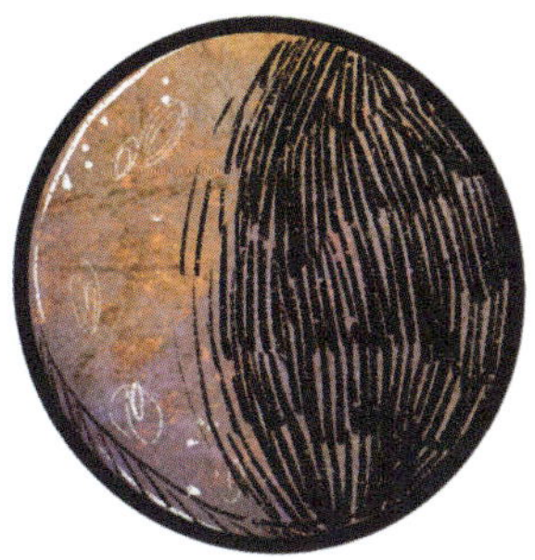

## *Waning Quarter Moon Remedy Blessing*

To be said over remedies while making them, during their brewing process, or before administering them:

*By the light of the quarter moon*
*wane and retire*
*release all troubles*
*all gloom and mire*

*as the moon turns inward*
*the remedy guides*
*to wisdom kept deep*
*between land and tide*

*blessed be*



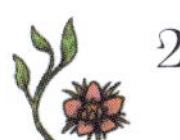

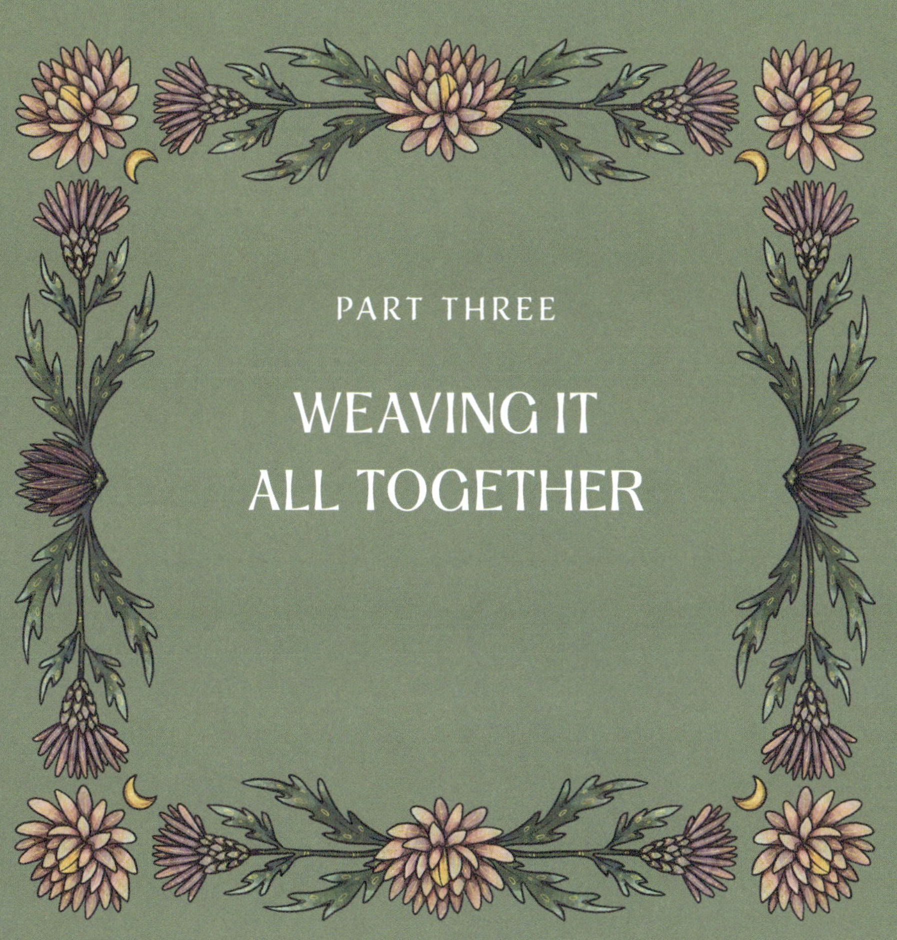

PART THREE

# WEAVING IT ALL TOGETHER

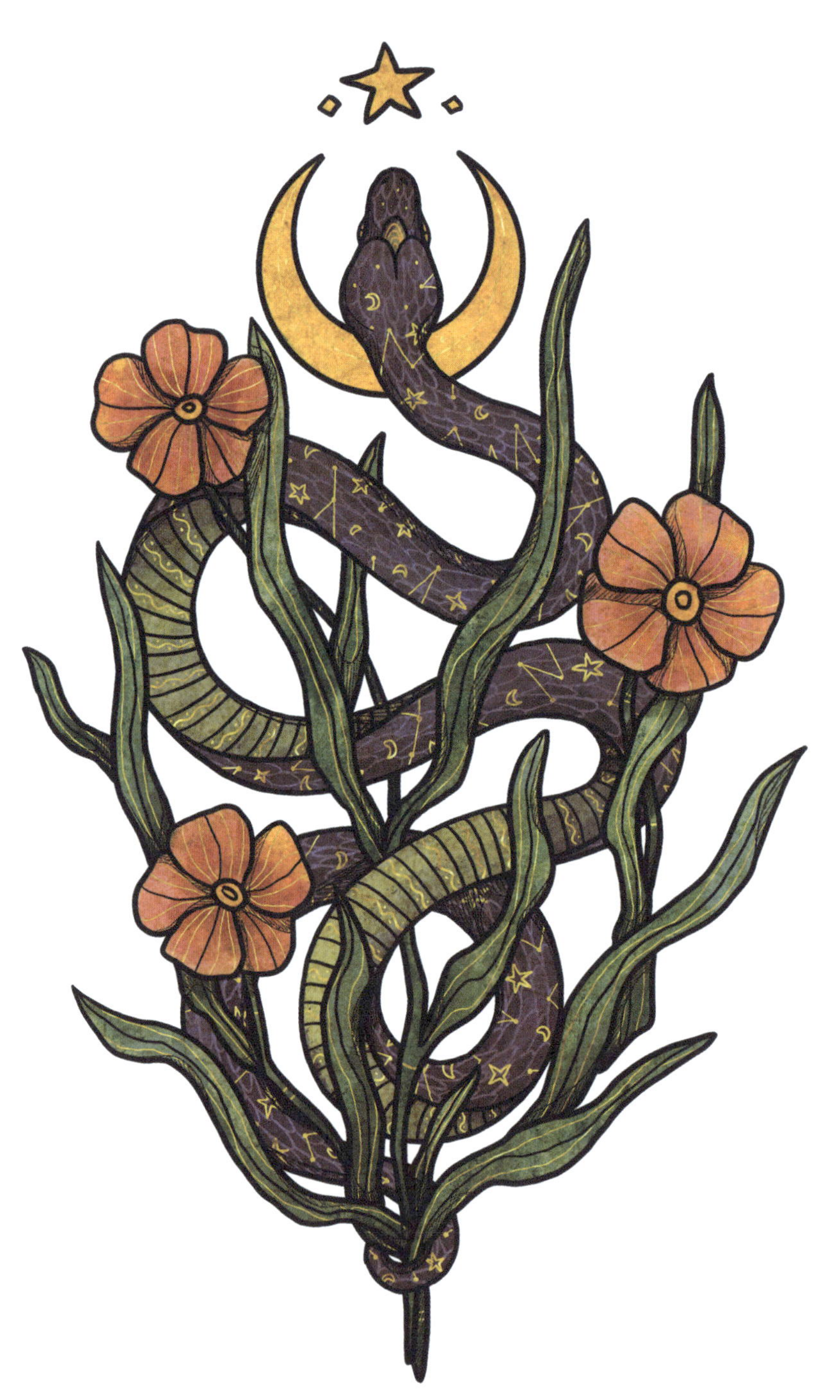

# When We Get Lost

At some point, you'll get lost. We all do. We fall off our path—or are pushed or lured by a siren song—tumbling from what feels comfortable and steady into someplace we'd rather not be. We are meant to get lost, lose our way, and find ourselves in the unfamiliar, but I don't believe we're meant to suffer in order to learn or have to pretend we have to go it alone. When we find ourselves dealing with anything from a slightly muffled sadness to deep traumas, our ability to feel connected to the land, at home in our bodies, or in loving relationships can seem unreliable or even entirely gone.

Years ago, I went through an intense burnout during which I had to slow down to what seemed like impossible stillness, realize I was lost, and let myself feel my way back home. I was lucky to have community support in finding the stories that needed telling, borrowing words until I could come up with my own and finding space to breathe and grieve while I began to explore and remap my inner world. Through this, I came to know the creature named grief I had avoided for so long. Slowly, slowly, grief transformed from a terrifying beast I felt ashamed about or worried would devour me into a steady companion I could set the table for, sit with, and then hold the door open for them to leave.

It is strange to be friends with something I know arises from something else falling apart, but learning to make space for grief meant I found out how to make space for grief's closest companions: compassion, love, and hope. When I hold open the door for grief, grief calls out in the night to their friends, many who have a long sky to cross but will eventually make it there by morning. So much of the complex healing needs I see arise from a sense of loss, whether loss of health, of loved ones, of connection, as well as disruptions to the grieving process. Plant allies like Hawthorn (*Crataegus monogyna*), Rose (*Rosa* spp.), Milky Oat (*Avena Sativa*), and Mugwort (*Artemisia vulgaris*) are some of the most powerful guides I know through the land of grief and emotional turmoil, and ones I've turned to again and again in my practice for myself or for my community.

What I learned with my own journey with grief, and with sitting with others, is that translation is an important part of healing: learning how to put the feelings in our bodies and the language of our experiences into words that can be understood by those we are in kinship with, whether friends, family, medical practitioners, and so on. Working with plant allies during this process helps us find the places of disruption within ourselves but still make it back to the surface. While all of us start with an initial pain from a wound or traumatic experience, the paths of healing are very different depending on whether you're surrounded by people who believe your pain and healing versus finding yourself unheard, dismissed, ignored, and isolated. As an herbalist, reaching for earth-centered language is the way I know how to help folks create the balm of words for their healing stories so that as they work with their plant allies and begin to settle into the rhythm of the year, they have plenty of words for their emerging myths.

When we begin from a place of knowing we already belong, finding our way back to the land that holds us, the relationships that heal us, and the inner wisdom that sustains us becomes less an act of triumphant willpower and luck, and instead an act of re-membering. We re-member—*put back together*—that we belong and work from there to find our pathways of kinship once again.

## Oldest of Herbs

One of the most powerful ways I know to re-member ourselves home to the land, our bodies, and our communities is turning to our plant ancestors, who provide us a more emotionally neutral space to connect with ancestral wisdom when we might struggle to do that with our own ancestral lines. Sometimes our families or cultures of origin are challenging to connect to in a way that feels healing or helpful. What I have learned working with plants as ancestors is there is always at least one ancestor—and often *many* more—who dreamed desperately of you and celebrates your existence. Working with plant allies as ancestors is one of the best ways I know of to find these beacons of benevolence within your ancestral lines.

I honor many herbs as ancestors in my practice from Rose (*Rosa* spp.) and Ginkgo (*Ginkgo biloba*), ancient plants present before our species evolved, to herbs that have been part of my ancestral lineage and cultural practices for


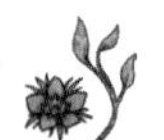

generations. Yet it was one plant, known as the "oldest of herbs," that drew me into honoring herbs as ancestors: Mugwort (*Artemisia* spp.).

The honorific "oldest of herbs" given to Mugwort comes from Anglo-Saxon lore, where it is celebrated for protecting against wounds, poisons, and any "foe who goes through the land."[26] What I have learned working with Mugwort is that it is incredibly good at moving emotions that have stagnated or frozen up in the body due to trauma. While most know Mugwort as a dreaming herb—which it most definitely is—it also has an amazing ability to move through time and space, traveling across our inner landscape to places we may have trouble accessing. Mugwort is excellent at unearthing stagnant energy and getting it to flow again, helping us find what may have been lost and reconnecting us to our dreaming selves as a way to draw us back home. Mugwort is a wayfinder, an old one who knows the path and a generous ally in healing work.

If you are feeling lost and don't know where to start, working with Mugwort can be a good place to begin. Mugwort can be worked with as a tea or tinctures, herbal oil or bath, burned as incense, carried in a charm bag, or used as a flower essence. Whether or not you work with Mugwort or another plant ancestor, I encourage you to open up to our plant allies less as a way to be fixed and more as a way to be found. The land never forgets, so let yourself be remembered.

## Mugwort Charm for Healing & Oracle Work

The following charm can be spoken over any remedy, used as a simple prayer, or said before working with your oracle map. I have started with a line from the Nine Herbs Charm of Anglo-Saxon tradition, but you can easily replace this with the name(s) of whatever plant ally you are working with.

*Mugwort, called Una,*
*oldest of herbs,*
*Where healing is needed*
*may it be known*
*Where the body is speaking*
*may it be heard*
*Where the land is calling*
*may it be felt*

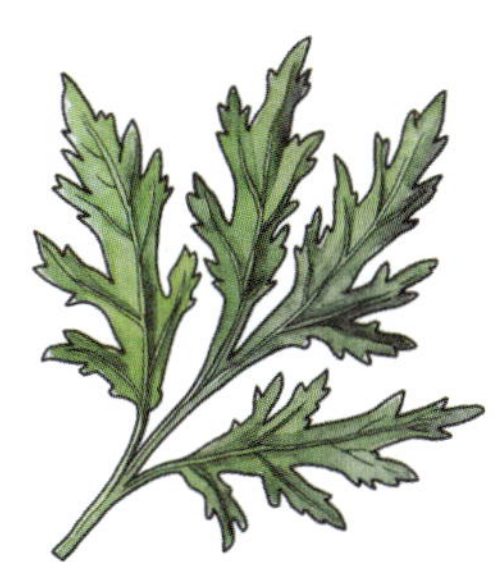

## Calling Life Back to the Land: Herbs for Restoring Vitality & Joy

Sometimes the world overcomes us and life feels heavy—the light that should uplift us instead seems too distant to bring comfort or far too bright and glaring. These are the times when we should seek out support, lean on our community, and go gently with ourselves. Plant allies can help us restore vitality, support our heart (see Opening Up, page 113), balance our body systems (see The Singing Land, page 70), and support brain health (see Waking Up from Winter, page 63), moving with us as we journey back to our joy.

**Eleuthero (*Eleutherococcus senticosus*):** Sometimes when we finally let ourselves slow down, our bodies tell us we need to rest deeper than we first expected. Eleuthero is a restorative adaptogen especially suited to helping folks recover from overwork. Indications include mental and physical burnout, low energy, poor memory and mental stamina, slow digestion.

**Linden (*Tilia x europaea*):** It may seem paradoxical, but sometimes our sadness stems from fearing our own tenderheartedness. Linden is one of those incredible allies reminding us it is through our tenderness we get to feel our way back home again to community and longevity. Indications for Linden include difficulty sleeping, signs of excess heat such as irritability, impatience, high blood pressure, heart palpitations caused by stress, and a general state of agitation.

**Milky Oat (*Avena sativa*):** Milky Oat is a foundational healer in my practice, offering the incredible gift of rebuilding the nervous system after a period of prolonged stress and depression. Indications include fatigue of all varieties, from chronic to adrenal to mental, brain fog, hormonal imbalance, menopause, low immunity, and recovering from illness.

**Rhodiola (*Rhodiola rosea*):** A useful adaptogen for depression, Rhodiola elevates our mood by increasing our serotonin and also addressing a number of depression-related symptoms like fatigue. Indications include low energy, chronic fatigue, low immunity, and burnout.


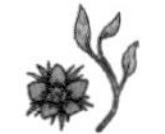

**Rosemary (*Salvia rosmarinus*):** Rosemary has a long record of use for memory, mental alertness, and "drying" an overly moist and cold brain, which is one way ancient herbalists described depression. I love how Rosemary moves energy and wakes up the body after a period of stagnation while combining well with herbs like Lemon Balm (*Melissa officinalis*) and Lavender (*Lavandula* spp.). Indications include overwork; depression arising from depleted mental, emotional, and physical resources; and feel unprotected in the world (combine with *Rosa* spp.).

## The Seeker's Oracle

This oracle map spread connects us with what we are seeking in our life and where the land within and around us is trying to draw our attention to. Choose six plant allies, whether the actual herb or a symbol:

one for your curious and seeking self looking for belonging
one for the land where you are being guided to
a plant ally to represent earth
a plant ally to represent air
a plant ally to represent fire
a plant ally to represent water

Prepare your space, brew a tea featuring one or more of your plant allies, and lay out your oracle of belonging. Ground and center, speaking any divining charms you wish to. When ready, take up your herbs or objects, close your eyes, and either toss or place them at random on the oracle map. For the seeker's oracle I like to hold the herbs to my heart, then to my lips where I whisper to them what I am seeking, then to my third eye before tossing the herbs or items onto the oracle map.

Where your curious and seeking self falls shows the place within you trying to get your attention and pull you toward belonging—pay attention to feelings, thoughts, and memories that might come up when you realize where this herb has landed. The position of the land herb indicates the area of your life the land around you is speaking most intensely through and pulling you toward as you go on your seeker's journey. The elemental places represent where you can draw on the energies of each to support you on your journey.

Let's say the plant ally of your curious and seeking self shows up in the area representing elderhood, perhaps drawing you to greater contemplation and planning for your later years. The land herbs shows up on the region for your sensory system, speaking of the land calling you to try relying more on your senses than your analytical mind on this next part of your journey. Finally, the earth herb and water herb land on the part of your oracle map for your skin, reinforcing the message of the land herb, while the fire herb lands at the place of your family, marking the importance of drawing energy from your connection to them, and the air herb lands at the place of your joints, encouraging flexibility and movement, to not get too stiff and stubborn on your journey.

From the oracle you might work with plant allies supporting vitality in the aging process, especially ones that are rich in smells, tastes, or other sensory experiences. Choose one to three herbs that help with adaptability, perhaps remind you of important familial connections and traditions, and strengthen the health of your skin.

## The Dark Moon

While there are no herbal correspondences within traditional western herbalism for the dark moon, it's a period of the lunar cycle I have a deep love for. The dark moon is a way to work with the energies of death and our feelings or even fears around it, as we contemplate the familiar suddenly disappearing, just like the dark moon disappears into the night. While I rarely make herbal medicine or work magick when the moon is dark, when I do they nearly always end up being some of my most beloved rites and remedies.

In my own lunar practice, I enjoy harvesting plants and making remedies that free up the dreaming body from being bound too tight to worldly expectation, helping release stagnant worries and heavy fears, settle unmoored energy, and make way for the lunar energy of the coming cycle.



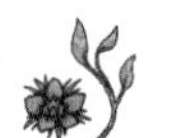

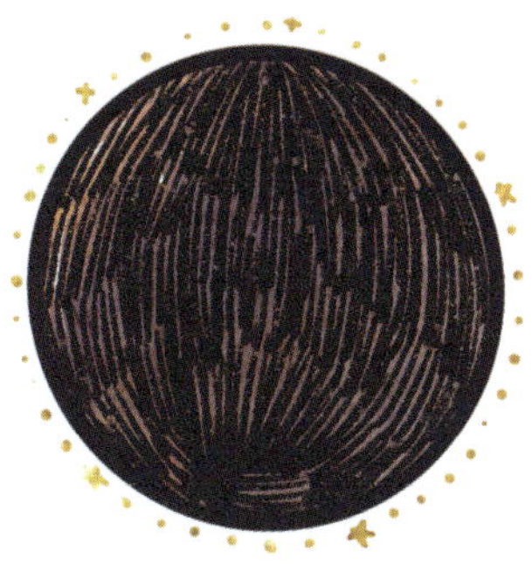

## Dark Moon Remedy Blessing

*By the shade of the dark moon*
*revel and rest*
*let worries decay*
*let untruths be redressed*

*as the moon takes to shadow*
*the remedy is bright*
*the stars dance the spiral*
*our/my magick takes flight*

*blessed be*

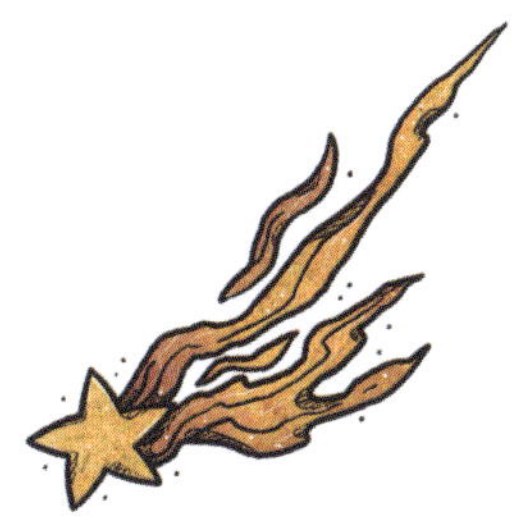

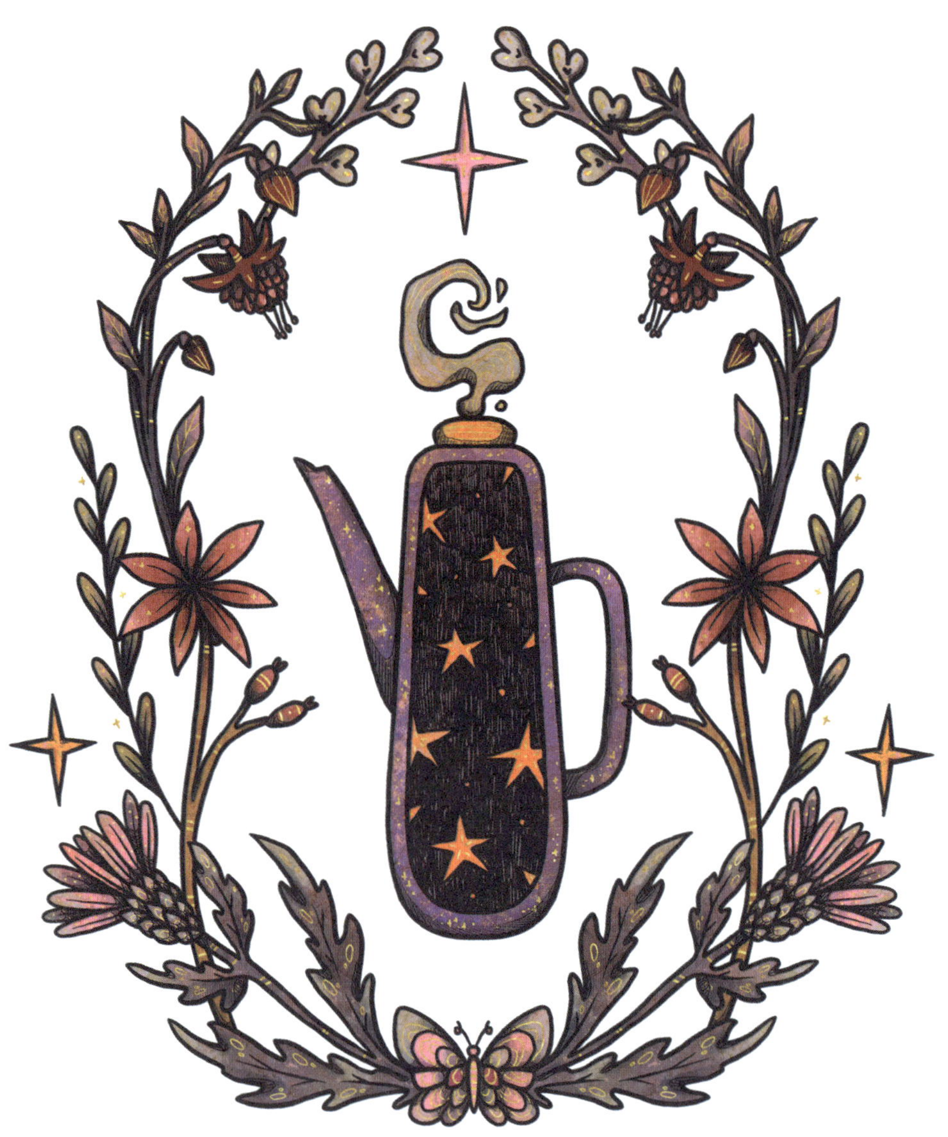

# *Belonging*

Developing your own apothecary of belonging is a practice of observation, engagement, and embodiment. We observe the land within and around us, expand our ability to perceive and be perceived, engage with what we find with intention, and embody our stories through ever-interconnected practices of kinship. It's time to put together all the practical knowledge, ritual suggestions, ways of thinking about the seasons, and ideas for cultivating community in a way that makes most sense to you, your sacred relationships, and the land you live with.

I invite you to go slowly and imagine what it is you might or might not want as part of your seasonal practices. It can be very easy, especially when we're inspired, to try and do *all the things*. Such enthusiasm is wonderful and will serve you best with just a little bit of discernment. It's important when creating an earth-centered practice in an age of intense marketing and culture-flattening algorithms to ask ourselves whenever we are drawn to a new pursuit whether we are trying to *develop* a practice or *buy* one. Each of us deserves to be held by our kinships and connections, so let yourself slow down, pause, mess around with, and create a practice that holds and inspires you.

My hope for you is a practice that feels comforting and sustainable like a well-worn blanket, easily mended, encompassing in its warmth, protective as a shelter, and multifunctional in its use. So let's start with the building blocks of life—the four elements moving through the land and weaving us all together.

## Begin with the Beginning

One of the easiest seasonal practices to start with is observing the elements of each season as they pass through the land around you. How do the elemental energies of earth—dense, stabilizing, and fertile—show up in spring? Or how does the elemental energy of fire, with its heat, brightness, and transformational movement, manifest throughout the land? Slowly, through expanding our perception of the world around and within us, seasons move from predominantly one thing to a series of micro-seasons and little climates throughout the weeks, days, and hours.

As we begin to notice the land through the seasons, we develop greater subtlety in what we are able to perceive and know. We can then pull that knowledge inward, bringing our developing skills to our inner landscape, starting to describe our experiences with simple elemental language like hot, cold, damp, and dry. We might notice, for example, that excess heat and tension arise within us when we have a stressful day and, just as a cool wind across the land lowers temperatures and pulls energy downward, so too can we choose cooling and relaxing remedies and activities to help our inner landscape feel at ease. With a seasonal practice we're not looking for heroic efforts in our everyday healing work, but simple adjustments that over time create resilient ways of being.

## Developing Kinship

We can bring these same elemental observations and actions to our relationships, learning how to reach for cooling and de-escalating techniques when things get overheated or energy-moving activities when things get stagnant. Relationships are complex, and being able to draw on the simple tools of an elemental foundation helps us ground and center as we work through their intricacies.

Alongside developing our skills of perception, we can start to cultivate our kinship skills with our plant allies. If you are new to or reconnecting with plant healing traditions, a beautiful place to start is working with one plant each season, allowing a bond to develop over time. Plant ally activities can include:

- Learning its medicinal use
- Exploring its folklore
- Creating remedies with it—a tea is a good place to start!
- Meditating with it, including observing where this plant appears in your inner landscape
- Paying attention to somatic experiences when working with it in remedy form or in ritual

- Engaging your senses with it
- Inviting it into your magickal work
- Incorporating it into food or drinks for meals and potlucks

Of course, we can expand any of these kinship activities to the land we live with starting with a tree in our neighborhood or sitting by the window and observing the sky every day. We can strengthen our kinship, too, by letting the borderlands of our inner landscape soften and shift, allowing greater connection with the lands of those we love and our communities. One of the simplest ways I know to develop kinship, especially with other humans, is to ask, *How can I share what I know?* This sharing is less about performing knowledge in order to receive praise and recognition, but offering what we know as an act of relationship-building and solidarity.

We can also ask ourselves, *How does this practice bring me back into community?* It took a long time for me to learn that getting enough rest and time to myself was essential for my ability to be in beloved community. So when I find myself falling into patterns of overwork, asking myself how I can get back to connecting with the land I live with and my relationships helps me slow down, sidestep unnecessary moralizing about what is "good" to do, and listen to the land within and around me. These are questions that are ever-asked and ever-answered, changing as we age and grow, showing up in new ways in our inner landscape.

## Creating Your Own Apothecary of Belonging

With your skills of observation engaged and kinship centered, you can begin to build your very own apothecary of belonging. On a practical level, an apothecary of belonging is a collection of seasonal remedies supporting the needs of our land-body in rhythm with the changing land around us. An apothecary of belonging is also the practices and skills to strengthen the ties of earth-centered kinship in your life, from seasonal celebrations to skill-sharing, sacred inquiry to easy rituals, and all the ways we know and are learning to call ourselves home again and again.

To develop your own apothecary of belonging, begin exploring your inner landscape and creating your own oracle map. From there you can choose an area of your life or healing concern to focus on for a full turning of the year. Let's say you want to strengthen your immune system after a long year of being sick—start by exploring seasonal plant allies to incorporate into your herbal practice. Check out Strengthening Boundaries(page 201) and identify one plant ally to work with. Begin with a single herb tea, a simple tincture, a one-herb bath, and stretch your remedy-making skills from there. Looking within, you can explore how this weakened immunity is showing up in your inner landscape, the elemental energetics and/or tissue states you feel connected to, and incorporate simple seasonal practices to rebuild your immunity.

Throughout the year you'll meet plant allies that work well for you and stock them in your apothecary, while recognizing how intertwined our inner landscapes and the land around us are and finding the practices that best support your seasonal ebb and flow. By starting slowly and simply, focusing on one primary plant ally each season, you'll have four plant allies you know well and can use in a variety of ways after a full turn of the wheel.

If you are an experienced practitioner, you can also consider the ways your practice is earth-centered, from how you make and/or acquire herbs to how you help your clients (re)develop kinship with the land, including exploring their inner landscapes. Learning more about how to craft an inclusive and inviting consultation or classroom is an important aspect of making space for lands to meet and mingle. As practitioners we can explore how our individual practices contribute to community health, as well as settle more deeply into our seasonal rhythms to protect against burnout and strengthen our resilient kinship. It can be really interesting to create an oracle map of your practice and use that alongside your personal oracle map to better understand the energy of your work each season.

Finally, I'm a big fan of the might-do list that allows us to dream big but make more space for joy than obligation. As you explore an herbal and magickal practice that is earth-based, kinship-centered, and seasonal in its rhythms, write down a list of what you *might do* each season. A spring might-do list could be full of everything from harvesting herbs to make oxymels to crafting your own


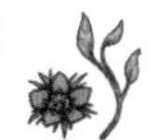

beeswax candles alongside community new moon rituals, but it is meant to inspire and remind you of the practices that make you feel whole, holy, and connected. You're not required to do anything but can allow yourself the freedom to maybe or maybe not do whatever you've thought of. I've found might-do lists wonderfully freeing in their obligationless enthusiasm and a great way to map out many paths to wherever you are being called each season.

Wherever your practice takes you, I hope you remember you are already a beloved of the land, a little land-body moving through time and space, and that your healing work creates an abundance of safe harbors, dry caves, and shade-rich forests for you to find shelter in and tend a fire for your community to gather round.

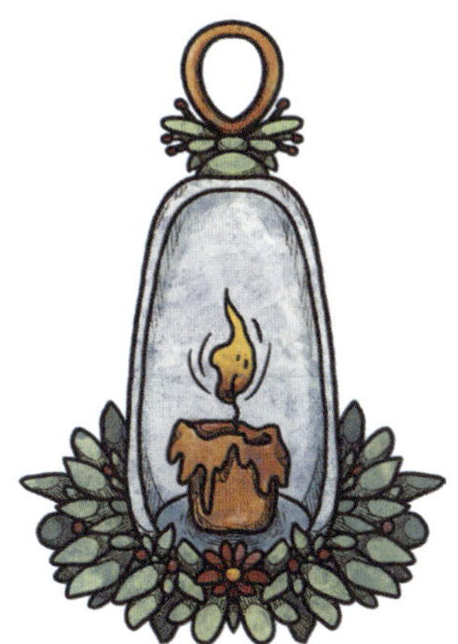

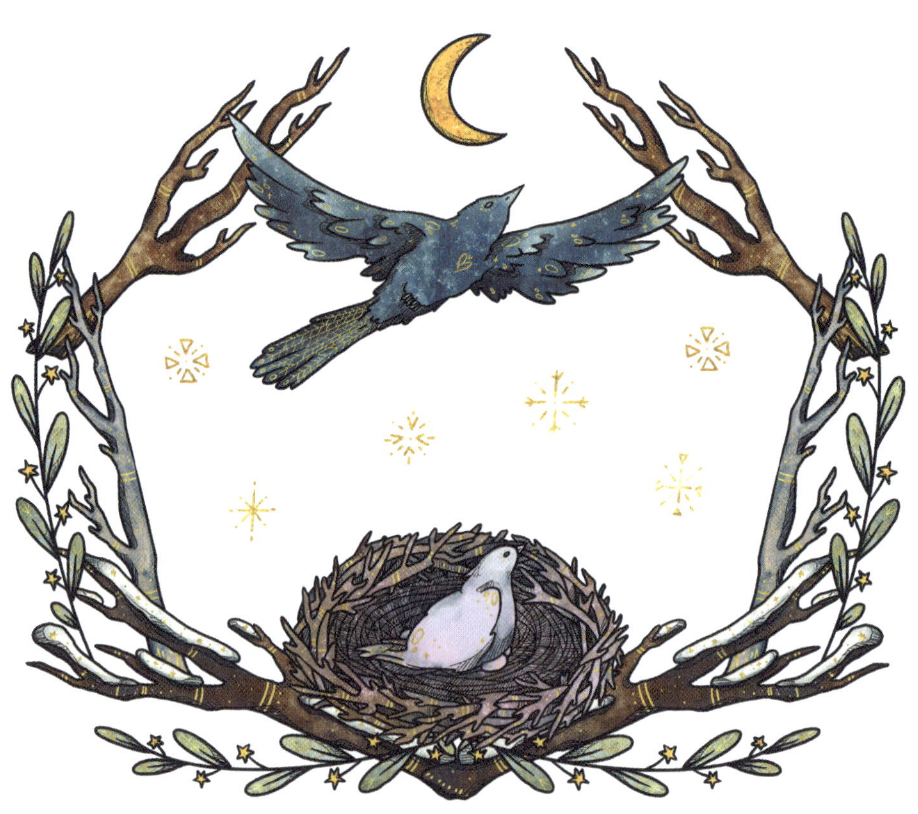

# Always Coming Home

A practice is like a river, changing us and changed by us as it flows through our lives, connecting us with the practices that have gone before and carrying knowledge to those who will come after. My hope is that by working with a current of practice ebbing and flowing through the seasons of the year, you'll find yourself in a place of embodied wisdom and carried by a coracle of kinship that lets you travel through the unfamiliar, the joyful, the uncomfortable, the sublime, and the transformative, ever protected against forgetting your own belonging. As rivers shape the land within us, so too can we shape our land-body with the rivers of our experiences, our desires, our hope, and our healing, creating an inner culture that supports and sustains us.

The world is uncertain (as it has always been), the times are interesting (as times were for our parents and grandparents and every generation before), and yet the path remains the same: The only way out is through; the only way home is with. While there is no practice, no spell, nor plant or remedy I know of that guards against all that may cause us pain, I know that pain is lessened when we reach for one another—our human and nonhuman kin and the land we all live with. The yearning and seeking, connecting and remembering we do through healing and magickal work are the rituals we practice in strange lands and unfamiliar times until we find ourselves home again.[27]

While writing this book, I've spent a fair amount of time under the shade of trees, and I've gotten to know the California scrub-jays that live in the urban woods of this lovely city. I've watched as they buried acorns during the warmer months to dig up again in winter. Then, come spring, their forgotten meals turn into Oak saplings sprouting up in all parts of the garden. I'm not quite sure how to describe the feeling that came over me when I realized what was happening—some hardness in me was undone knowing these noisy, funny, and wildly intelligent birds were planting forests, continuing the traditions of their ancestors, providing shade and habitat for generations to come. As I was tangled up in my own thoughts and fears of what it was to write something so permanent as a book—not knowing if I was up to the task or worthy, much less how my words would be read or intentions understood—I found myself weeping at Oak saplings as squirrels chittered at me from Redwood branches, suddenly less afraid of the mystery ahead when met with the power of a precariously made but enduring forest of jays.

Part of the practice of belonging is letting yourself be seen with all your discomfort and confusion alongside all of the love and relief that comes from being perceived as whole and holy. So I plant my acorns, remembering where many of them lie in the land to dig up again when times are thin and sustenance is needed, but also realizing I'll forget plenty of them, not knowing what they might become. I hope that some become long-lived Oaks, but mostly I hope that this work of mine has inspired your own practice of planting seeds like offerings, letting the land within, around, and between us grow them into future forests of mirth and reverence. Together may we create a deep shade of kinship that shelters for generations, where we always know that we belong.

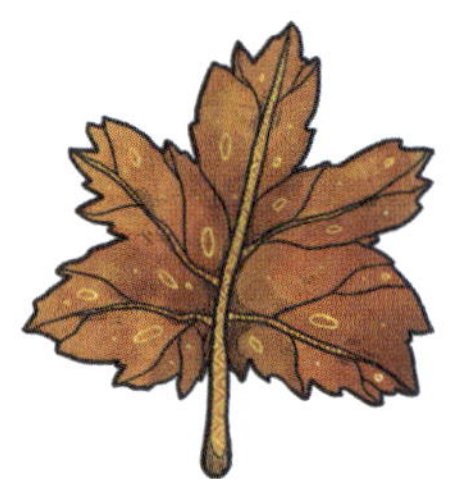

# Appendixes

## Standard Dosage

In traditional western herbalism, many of us operate within the guidelines of "standard dosage" when recommending how much of an herb should be taken over the course of the day. If you are on medication or have complex medical needs, you should work with an herbalist to determine the best dosage guidelines for you.

**Infusions (Tea & Decoctions):** A generous teaspoon (25 g) of dried herb per 8 oz. of water for infusions or 1 heaping tablespoon per 8 oz. for decoctions up to three times daily for chronic conditions and up to six times daily for acute conditions. Use twice as much with fresh herbs.

**Extracts (Tinctures & Glycerites):** For adults, 20–60 drops (about 1–2 dropperfuls) up to three times daily for chronic conditions and up to six times daily for acute conditions. For children 6–12 years in age, generally 10–30 drops up to four times daily. For toddlers, 5–15 drops up to three times daily and babies 3–5 drops up to three times daily, but I recommended looking up and using weight-to-dosage guidelines for pediatric doses (often listed on tincture bottles themselves, but, if not, they can be easily found in trusted *materia medica*). Tinctures are most enjoyable mixed in water or juice. For the young, tinctures can also be used in baths, washes, and compresses.

**Syrups:** ½ teaspoon to 1 tablespoon, three to four times per day for chronic conditions and every few hours for acute conditions.

**Tablets & Capsules:** 1–2 size 0 capsules or 1 of the 00 capsules up to three times daily.

**Powders:** ½ teaspoon–1 tablespoon powder up to three times daily.

**Flower Essences:** 1–3 drops taken directly under the tongue, in a glass of water or rubbed into the skin up to three times daily or as needed.

## *A Low-Dosage Variation*

As I work with a lot of sensitive folks, I tend to scale down standard dosage recommendations in most chronic health cases, specifically with extracts. Instead, I use low-dosage guidelines, which are sometimes known as drop dosages. These low dosages are based in tradition and were a common way of recommending herbs within traditional western herbalism. For most folks, especially sensitive folks looking to take herbs on a restorative basis over a long period, low and drop dosages are very effective.

For acute conditions, I follow the higher amounts recommended by standard dosage.

**Extracts (Tinctures & Glycerites):** 1–10 drops of tincture or glycerite taken up to three times daily. For chronic health concerns with children under 12, I often recommend no more than 5 drops up to three times daily.

Additionally, I was taught that when working with herbs over an extended period of time (i.e., three months or longer), take them for three consecutive weeks and then break for one week. I enjoy this cycle as a helpful way of gently checking in with your body every few weeks about what it needs and any adjustments to make to your herbal practice.

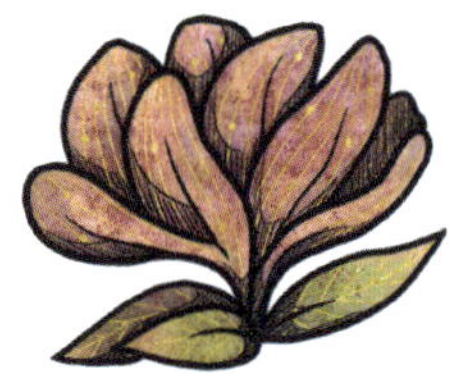

## A Quick Guide to Folk-Style Remedy-Making

Remedy-making in traditional western herbalism can be highly technical, but it can also be done through much simpler folk techniques. The following provides brief descriptions for making a variety of common remedies via folk techniques from the most commonly used to the least, but you should always reference your *materia medica* when determining the best method for preparing a particular plant.

**Tea (Standard dosage for daily use):** Use standard dosage and brew for fifteen to twenty minutes. Store refrigerated and use within three days.

**Tea (Medicinal dosage for acute symptoms):** Use standard dosage and brew at least thirty minutes, preferably longer. Store refrigerated and use within three days.

**Tea (Bath):** Brew 1 cup of herbs in a quart of water for at least twenty minutes. Strain and add to bathwater.

**Decoction:** 1 heaping tbsp of herbs per cup of water. Add herbs to water in a saucepan and bring to a boil. Low simmer for fifteen to twenty minutes, remove from heat, let sit another hour. Strain and drink. Store refrigerated and use within three days.

**Extract (Alcohol):** Prepare dried or fresh plant material by grinding into fine pieces. Place plant material in a glass container and cover with alcohol (80–190 proof) so that there is 1 inch of alcohol floating above or below plant material. Add a dash of water, seal jar with airtight lid, and brew for a full cycle of the moon, shaking daily. After a full lunar cycle, strain out plant material and bottle. Will have a three-plus-year shelf life if stored in a cool, dark place.

**Extract (Nonalcoholic):** Prepare plant material as with an alcohol extract. Add vegetable glycerin or raw apple cider vinegar instead of alcohol, adding no water if the plant is fresh and only a small dash if plant material is dried. Brew as above. Has one- to two-year shelf life for glycerites and three-plus-years for vinegars.

**Liniment:** Prepare, brew, and strain plant material as an extract using either vodka or witch hazel extract as base. Use topically, with or without essential oils, for strains, pains, swellings, etc. Has three-plus-year shelf life.

**Herbal Oil:** Prepare dried to partially dried plant material by grinding into small pieces. Cover plant material with oil of choice (Olive, Coconut, Sweet Almond, and Jojoba are good choices) with an inch of liquid above or below plant material. After a full lunar cycle, strain out plant material and bottle. Use topically as needed. Has six-month to one-year shelf life if stored in a cool, dark place.

**Salve:** Mix prepared 4 parts herbal oil with 1 part wax (beeswax or candelilla) for a firmer salve or a 5:1 oil to wax ratio for a softer one. Melt wax into oil with a double boiler; pour into containers and let firm. Has six-month to two-year shelf life if stored in a cool, dark place.

**Powder**: Grind plant material and use a fine tea strainer to sift out larger pieces. Store in cool, dark space, preferably the fridge, and use within six to nine months.

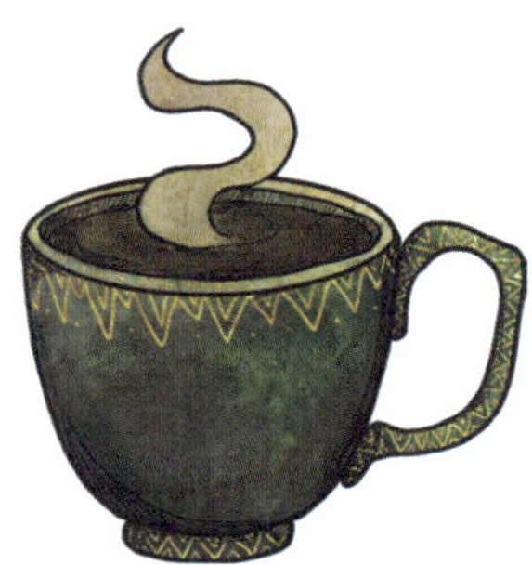

# Contraindications

Most of the herbs included in *The Apothecary of Belonging* are generally considered safe for all age groups, but while this contraindications list is a good place to start, you should always cross-reference your trusted *materia medica* or work with an herbalist to determine which herbs are best for you, especially if you are on any type of medication, are pregnant or lactating, or have complex medical needs.

**Aloe Vera (*Aloe barbadensis/Aloe vera*):** Contraindicated during pregnancy, however, the contraindication usually refers to the outer, yellow latex of the leaf.

**Angelica (*Angelica archangelica*):** Not for use in pregnancy and by those with bleeding disorders (including menorrhagia), Gastroesophageal Reflux Disease (GERD), reflux, peptic ulcers, hypertension, and salicylate sensitivity. Avoid a week prior to surgery. Use with caution with diabetics as the plant can increase blood sugar levels.

**Ashwagandha (*Withania somnifera*):** Use only in the late third trimester in pregnancy with practitioner supervision. Caution with diabetics—monitor blood glucose—and with thyroid medication.

**Basil, Sweet & Holy (*Ocimum* spp.):** Generally regarded as safe. There are contradictory animal studies regarding whether or not the herb is safe during pregnancy (it is used within Ayurvedic tradition during pregnancy)—avoid or consult with a practitioner. It may have antifertility qualities. Use caution with diabetes and blood glucose levels. Avoid with anticoagulants and thyroid medication.

**Black Cohosh (*Actaea racemosa*):** Avoid during pregnancy, lactation, and for children under twelve. May interfere with oral contraceptives.

**Boneset (*Eupatorium perfoliatum*):** Large doses can lead to vomiting and diarrhea. Use no more than five days consecutively and then take a break.

**Borage (*Borago officinalis*):** Avoid during pregnancy. Avoid with anticoagulants and stop usage a week before surgery. Best used in the short-term.

**Burdock (*Arctium lappa*):** Avoid use during the first trimester of pregnancy, but other herbalists recommend avoiding it throughout all trimesters and during lactation, so consult with a practitioner. Avoid with insulin and other hypoglycemic medications.

**Butterbur (*Petasites hybridus*):** Avoid during pregnancy and lactation.

**Calendula (*Calendula officinalis*):** Generally regarded as safe, but avoid during pregnancy because of emmenagogue qualities. Caution with sedatives and insulin/hypoglycemic medications.

**California Poppy (*Eschscholzia californica*):** Avoid during pregnancy and lactation. Contraindicated in glaucoma. Avoid if on monoamine oxidase inhibitors (MAOIs).

**Catnip (*Nepeta cataria*):** Avoid during pregnancy. Short periods (no more than a week or two) and small doses are appropriate for young ones.

**Chamomile (*Matricaria chamomilla*):** Contraindicated for folks with ragweed allergies. Some experience contact dermatitis with the fresh plant. Avoid with anticoagulant medications.

**Chickweed (*Stellaria media*):** Generally regarded as safe.

**Cleavers (*Galium aparine*):** Generally regarded as safe.

**Cramp Bark (*Viburnum opulus*):** The uncooked berries are toxic. Avoid in cases of salicylate allergy, hypotension, kidney stones, and bleeding disorders. Stop use a week before surgery.

**Damiana (*Turnera diffusa*):** Avoid during pregnancy and lactation. May interfere with iron absorption. Caution with diabetes medication due to Damiana's effect on blood sugar.

**Dandelion (*Taraxacum officinale*):** Contact with the fresh latex may cause contact dermatitis in certain individuals (very rare). Contraindicated in bile duct obstruction, acute gallbladder inflammation, acute gastrointestinal inflammation, and intestinal blockage. Use caution with diuretics and hypotensive medication.


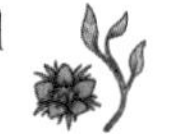

**Echinacea (*Echinacea purpurea*):** Avoid with ragweed allergies. May decrease effectiveness of immunosuppressant medicines.

**Elder (*Sambucus nigra*):** Generally regarded as safe.

**Elecampane (*Inula helenium*):** Avoid during pregnancy and lactation. Large doses may cause gastric spasms, vomiting, diarrhea, and allergic hypersensitivity.

**Eleuthero (*Eleutherococcus senticosus*):** For pregnancy and lactation there are contradictory recommendations, so I advise working with a practitioner who can supervise and support.

**Eyebright (*Euphrasia officinalis*):** Generally considered safe.

**Fennel (*Foeniculum vulgare*):** Avoid or only use in small doses during early pregnancy.

**Garlic (*Allium sativum*):** Avoid large doses in pregnancy. Caution with GI issues and with anticoagulants.

**Ginger (*Zingiber officinale*):** Low doses in pregnancy. Avoid in cases of peptic ulcers and hyperacidity. Caution with anticoagulant drugs.

**Ginkgo (*Ginkgo biloba*):** Caution with bleeding disorders and anticoagulants, MAOIs, and insulin. Discontinue use a week before surgery.

**Goldenrod (*Solidago* spp.):** Avoid with edema, diuretics, and antihypertensives.

**Gotu Kola (*Centella asiatica*):** Caution during pregnancy—use with support from a practitioner. Large doses can cause vertigo and headache. Avoid for overactive thyroid conditions. Avoid with barbiturates and insulin/hypoglycemic and cholesterol-lowering medications. Caution with depressants such as alcohol and opiates.

**Hawthorn (*Crataegus monogyna*):** Use with caution with heart medications, bleeding disorders, and hypotension. Caution with anticoagulants, hypotensives, CNS depressants, insulin, and vasodilators.

**Holy Basil (*Ocimum tenuiflorum*):** See *Basil*.

**Hyssop (*Hyssopus officinalis*):** Avoid during pregnancy.

**Lady's Mantle (*Alchemilla vulgaris*):** Avoid in pregnancy (but can be used right before labor to help prevent postpartum hemorrhage).

**Lavender (*Lavandula* spp.):** Generally considered safe.

**Lemon Balm (*Melissa officinalis*):** May interfere with thyroid medications. Avoid in cases of glaucoma as Lemon Balm may increase eye pressure.

**Licorice (*Glycyrrhiza glabra*):** Avoid during pregnancy. Avoid in large amounts and use for a short time period. Caution with many pharmaceutical medications, so work with an herbal practitioner if you use any.

**Linden (*Tilia x europaea*):** Generally considered safe.

**Lomatium (*Lomatium dissectum*):** Low dosage recommended. Avoid use during pregnancy and lactation.

**Marshmallow (*Althea officinalis*):** Generally considered safe.

**Meadowsweet (*Filipendula ulmaria*):** Avoid in cases of salicylate allergy, asthma, and bleeding disorders. Avoid with anticoagulants. Caution during pregnancy and lactation.

**Milk Thistle (*Silybum marianum*):** Avoid with daisy (*Asteraceae*) family allergy. Avoid with insulin and hypoglycemic medication.

**Milky Oat (*Avena sativa*):** Generally considered safe.

**Motherwort (*Leonurus cardiaca*):** Avoid during pregnancy and lactation. Do not use in cases of menorrhagia. Use only in the last part of pregnancy with supervision of an herbalist as it can start labor.

**Mugwort (*Artemisia vulgaris*):** Best for short-term use (no more than a month at a time without a break).

**Mullein (*Verbascum thapsus*):** Generally regarded as safe.



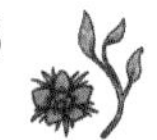

**Myrrh (*Commiphora molmol*):** Avoid in pregnancy and lactation. Avoid in cases of autoimmune disease, acute kidney infections, and menorrhagia. Short-term use only.

**Nettles (*Urtica dioica*):** Nettle leaf is generally considered safe. Do not take the root during pregnancy.

**Ocotillo (*Fouquieria splendens*):** Avoid during pregnancy.

**Oregano (*Oregano vulgaris*):** Avoid during pregnancy.

**Passionflower (*Passiflora incarnata*):** Avoid large doses during pregnancy, though smaller doses are generally considered safe. Do not consume unripe fruits as they can be toxic.

**Peppermint (*Mentha piperita*):** Avoid large amounts during lactation as mints may dry up the milk supply, but can be used in small amounts for mastitis.

**Plantain (*Plantago major/Plantago lanceolata*):** Generally regarded as safe. Caution with anticoagulants.

**Raspberry Leaf (*Rubus idaeus*):** Generally regarded as safe but caution in early pregnancy.

**Red Clover (*Trifolium pratense*):** Avoid with blood thinner medication or if you have a bleeding disorder. Avoid at least a week before surgery. Use during pregnancy and lactation only in small doses with guidance from an herbal practitioner.

**Reishi (*Ganoderma lucidum*):** Generally considered safe, but use with guidance from an herbal practitioner during pregnancy and lactation. Avoid if you have mushroom or mold allergies. Discontinue a week before surgery.

**Rhodiola (*Rhodiola rosea*):** Take at a time different from mineral supplements.

**Rose (*Rosa* spp.):** Generally considered safe.

**Rosemary (*Salvia rosmarinus*):** Generally considered safe but avoid large doses and taking with mineral supplements. Avoid during pregnancy (as food seasoning is fine).

**Sage (*Salvia officinalis*):** Avoid large doses during pregnancy. Avoid while lactating as it dries up milk. In large doses, its thujone content may adversely affect those with epilepsy, high blood pressure, or kidney disease.

**Saw Palmetto (*Serenoa repens*):** Avoid during pregnancy. Avoid in bleeding disorders and with anticoagulants. Discontinue a week before surgery.

**Schisandra (*Schisandra chinensis*):** Avoid during early pregnancy and later only use with practitioner guidance. Not for children under two. Avoid in cases of excess heat like fever and acute infections. Traditional Chinese Medicine warns against use during early stages of cough and rash.

**Self-Heal (*Prunella vulgaris*):** Generally considered safe but avoid with insulin and hypoglycemic medications.

**Shatavari (*Asparagus racemosus*):** Avoid in cases of diarrhea, acute lung congestion, acid reflux, gastritis, cystic breast issues, cholestasis, and excess damp and cold.

**Skullcap (*Scutellaria lateriflora*):** Generally considered safe. Mixed recommendations for during pregnancy, so consult with your herbalist.

**Spilanthes (*Spilanthes oleracea*):** Avoid during pregnancy and lactation.

**St. Joan's Wort (*Hypericum perforatum*):** Do not combine with antidepressants or any pharmaceutical drug without supervision from a health practitioner (use flower essence instead). Avoid during pregnancy or while nursing. Not for children two and under.

**Thyme (*Thymus vulgaris*):** Generally regarded as safe but avoid large amounts during pregnancy.

**Turmeric (*Curcuma longa*):** While safe in food, Turmeric should be used with caution during pregnancy. Avoid with jaundice, acute hepatitis, bleeding disorders, hyperacidity, peptic ulcers.

**Uva Ursi (*Arctostaphylos uva-ursi*):** Avoid during pregnancy and lactation. Avoid in cases of hypoglycemia, kidney disease, and inflammatory intestinal conditions.


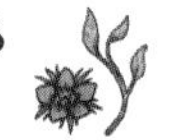

Not for use with children under twelve. Short-term use recommended (one month or less).

**Valerian (*Valeriana* spp.):** Use with caution and in low doses, if at all, during pregnancy. Not for young children. Best in low doses as high dosages can be overly sedating, resulting in lethargy, depression, nausea, headache, and dizziness. Avoid with cental nervous system (CNS) depressants including alcohol, opiates, benzodiazepines, anesthetics, tricyclic antidepressants, antiepileptics. Discontinue a week before surgery.

**Vervain (*Verbena* spp.):** Do not use during pregnancy. Do not take at the same time with mineral supplements. Avoid with anticoagulants.

**Vitex (*Vitex agnus-castus*):** Avoid during pregnancy. Avoid with estrogen-sensitive cancers.

**White Willow Bark (*Salix alba*):** Do not use if you have an aspirin allergy. Do not use for viral infection, such as influenza or chicken pox, with children under the age of sixteen to avoid Reye syndrome. Avoid use with bleeding disorders or anticoagulants, barbiturates, or sedatives.

**Wood Betony (*Betonica officinalis*):** Avoid during pregnancy and nursing. Caution with hypotensive and antidiabetic medications. High doses may cause intestinal upset, including cramping, gas, nausea, and diarrhea.

**Yarrow (*Achillea millefolium*):** Avoid large doses during pregnancy as Yarrow can act like a uterine stimulant. Caution with epileptic patients. Very large doses can cause headaches.

**Yellow Dock (*Rumex crispus*):** Avoid during pregnancy and lactation. Avoid with kidney issues, including kidney stones. Short-term use only.

**Yerba Santa (*Eriodictyon californicum*):** Generally considered safe, but caution during pregnancy.



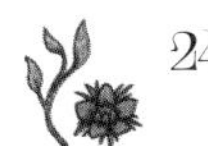

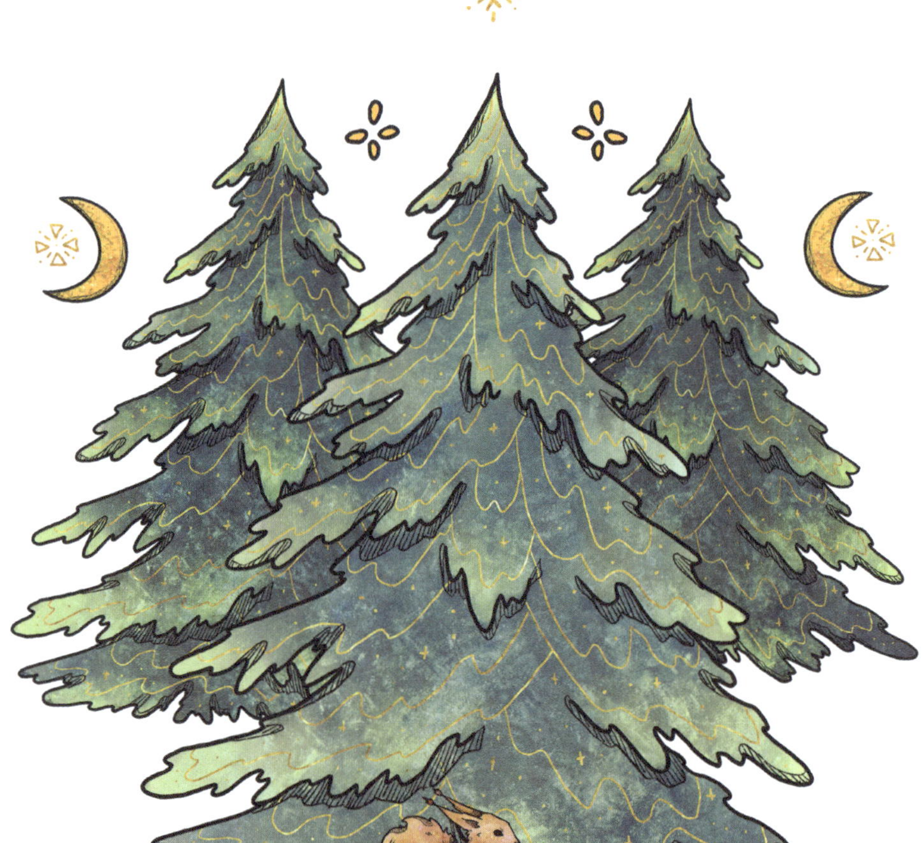

# Acknowledgments

A heartfelt thanks to the folks at Weiser who offered me the chance to write a book before I knew what I wanted to write and then trusted me when I figured it out.

To Julie James—my first herb teacher who set the standard for all to come. To Beth Maiden—the seeds of this book were born in the community spaces you created. To those I've sat in circle with and learned from—a deep well of gratitude. To my students—thank you for helping me become the teacher who could write this book for you.

To Madeleine—ever delighted as I struggled to name my feelings beyond "something akin to moss." I cried when we first met because of how kind and wise you are—I'm still weeping (*joyfully, mossily*).

To Grammy and Grandpa—for teaching me about shelter by making such a steadfast one for me to grow up in. To my parents—who celebrated my earliest writing and terribly earnest poetry. To my brother—my first reason to learn and model hope —how lucky I am to be your big sister.

To Tel—who I would call my rock, but I think you're something more precious and enduring. And to my daughters—I am in constant awe and joy for all that you are becoming. *I love you so much.*

To the land, my ancestors, my beloved kin—all begins and ends and begins again with you.

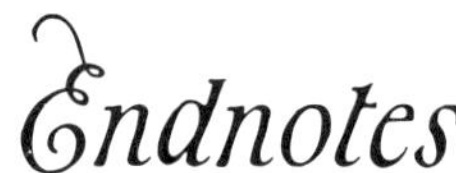

# Endnotes


1 J. S. Hopkins, "Nigon wyrta galdor, popularly known as the Nine Herbs Charm: a new annotated and illustrated translation," 2020, *mimisbrunnr.info* (accessed July 2022).

2 Thomas Bartram, *Bartram's Encyclopedia of Herbal Medicine* (London: Constable & Robinson Ltd, 1998), 48.

3 Mary Siisip Geniusz, *Plants Have So Much to Give Us, All We Have to Do Is Ask: Anishinaabe Botanical Teachings* (Minneapolis: University of Minnesota Press, 2015), 205–6.

4 Paul Beyerl, *A Compendium of Herbal Magick* (Custer, WA: Phoenix Publishing, 1998), 313.

5 Karen M. Rose, *The Art & Practice of Spiritual Herbalism: Transform, Heal & Remember with the Power of Plants and Ancestral Medicine* (Beverly, MA: Quarto Publishing, 2022), 156.

6 Thanks, Silver RavenWolf.

7 Brigitte Mars, *The Desktop Guide to Herbal Medicine* (Laguna Beach, CA: Basic Health Publications, 2007), 73.

8 Scott Cunningham, *Cunningham's Encyclopedia of Magical Herbs* (St. Paul, MN: Llewellyn, 2001), 169.

9 Cunningham, 169.

10 Stephen Taylor, *The Humoral Herbal: A Practical Guide to the Western Energetic System of Health, Lifestyle, and Herbs* (London: Aeon Books, 2021), 322.

11 Hildegard von Bingen, *Hildegard's Healing Plants: From Her Medieval Classic "Physica,"* trans. Bruce W. Hozeski (Boston: Beacon Press, 2001), 7.

12 Mars, *The Desktop Guide to Herbal Medicine*, 212.

13 Taylor, *The Humoral Herbal*, 353.

14 Mars, *The Desktop Guide to Herbal Medicine*, 159.

15 Judith Berger, *Herbal Rituals* (New York: St. Martin's Press, 1998), 134.

16 Hildegard von Bingen, *Hildegard's Healing Plants*, 115.

17 Geniusz, *Plants Have So Much to Give Us, All We Have to Do Is Ask*, 188.

18 Val Thomas, "The Nine Herbs Charm: Plants Poisons and Poetry," Herbal History Research Network, February 11, 2021, *herbalhistory.org* (accessed July 2022).

19 Bartram, *Bartram's Encyclopedia of Herbal Medicine*, 341.

20 Deb Soule, *The Roots of Healing: A Woman's Book of Herbs* (New York: Citadel Press, 1995), 159.

21 Cunningham, *Cunningham's Encyclopedia of Magical Herbs*, 207.

22 Mars, *The Desktop Guide to Herbal Medicine*, 123.

23 Plot twist: Thyme probably wasn't in the original recipe.

24 Rose, , *The Art & Practice of Spiritual Herbalism*, 42.

25 Rose, 42.

26 Hopkins, "Nigon wyrta galdor, popularly known as the Nine Herbs Charm."

27 Go and read the Initiation Song by Ursula K. LeGuin in *Always Coming Home* (Berkeley: University of California Press, 2001) for a blessing on your journey.




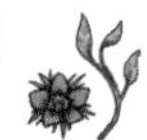

# Index

## D



## E



## F



## G



## H




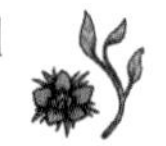

## R



## S

## T



## U



## V



## W



## X–Y–Z

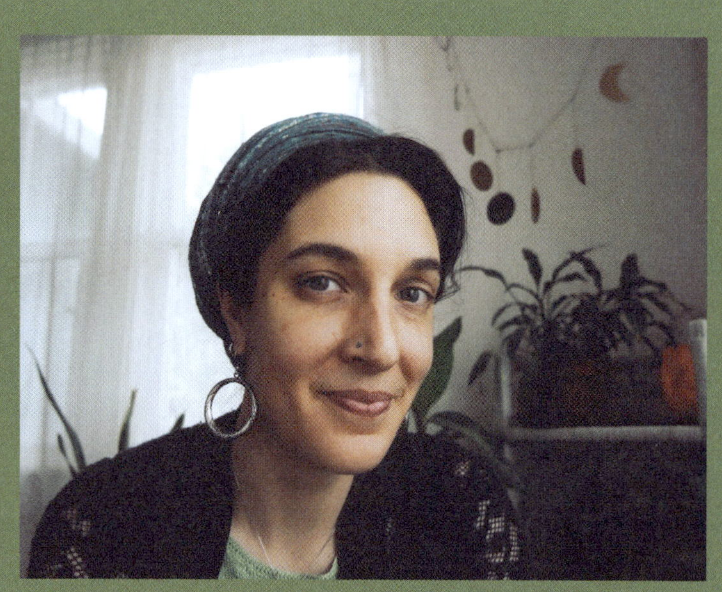

# About the Author

Alexis J. Cunningfolk (she/they) is a community herbalist and witch whose work is centered in the values of embodiment, kinship, and a curiosity that liberates. Led by a childhood interest in herbalism and magickal practice to found Worts & Cunning Apothecary in 2010, Alexis's intersectionality and love for creating spaces of belonging are born of her lived experience as a lesbian, a woman of mixed ancestry, and a third-culture kid. Her work has led her around the country, presenting at various magickal, herbal, and academic conferences, as well as facilitating rituals ranging from a handful of folks to hundreds. She offers much of her work for free or low cost, wild seeding wisdom as an act of gratitude and spell of collective liberation. Find her work at *wortsandcunning.com*.

# *To Our Readers*

Weiser Books, an imprint of Red Wheel/Weiser, publishes books across the entire spectrum of occult, esoteric, speculative, and New Age subjects. Our mission is to publish quality books that will make a difference in people's lives without advocating any one particular path or field of study. We value the integrity, originality, and depth of knowledge of our authors.

Our readers are our most important resource, and we appreciate your input, suggestions, and ideas about what you would like to see published.

Visit our website at *www.redwheelweiser.com*, where you can learn about our upcoming books and free downloads, and also find links to sign up for our newsletter and exclusive offers.

You can also contact us at *info@rwwbooks.com* or at

Red Wheel/Weiser, LLC
65 Parker Street, Suite 7
Newburyport, MA 01950

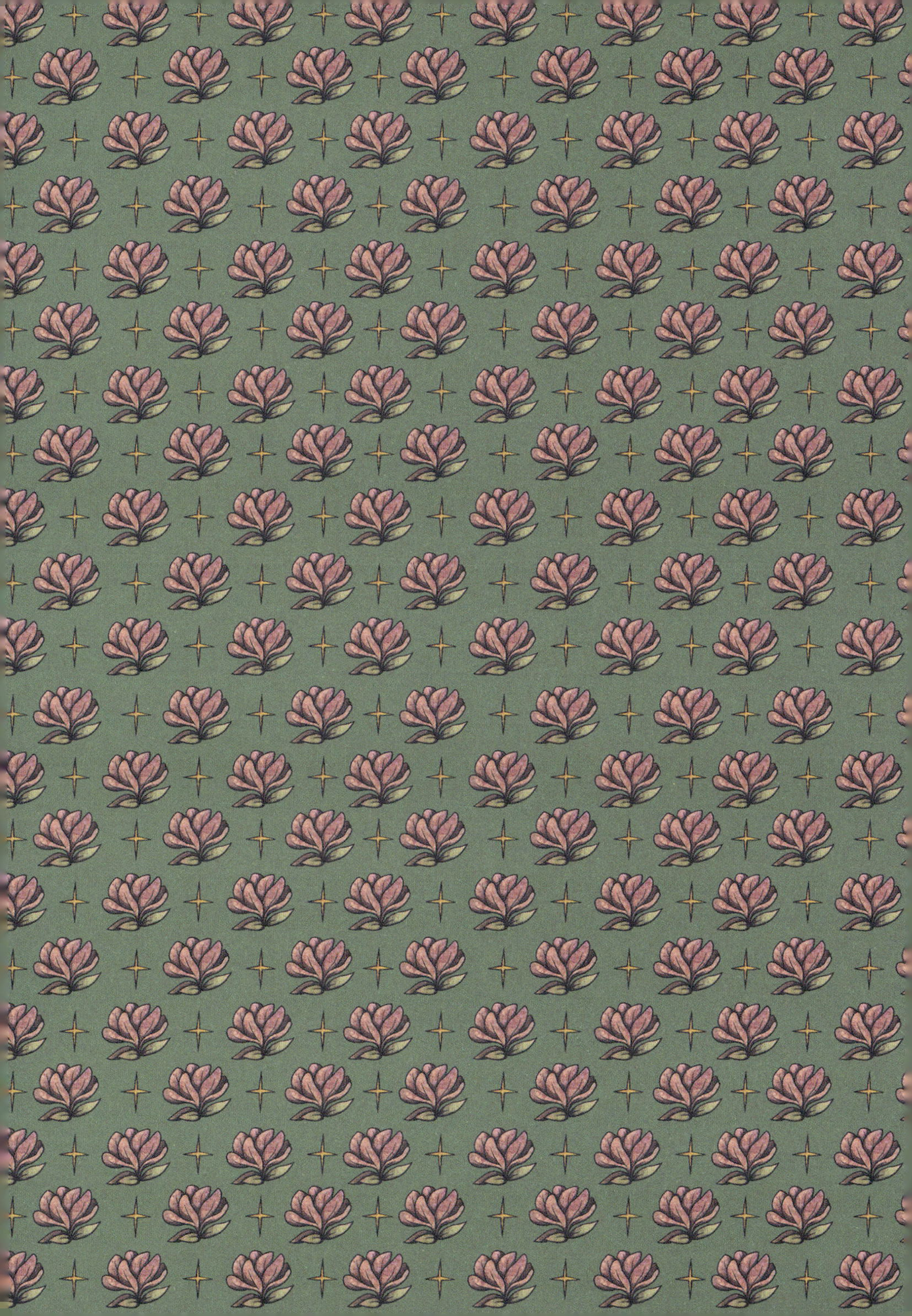

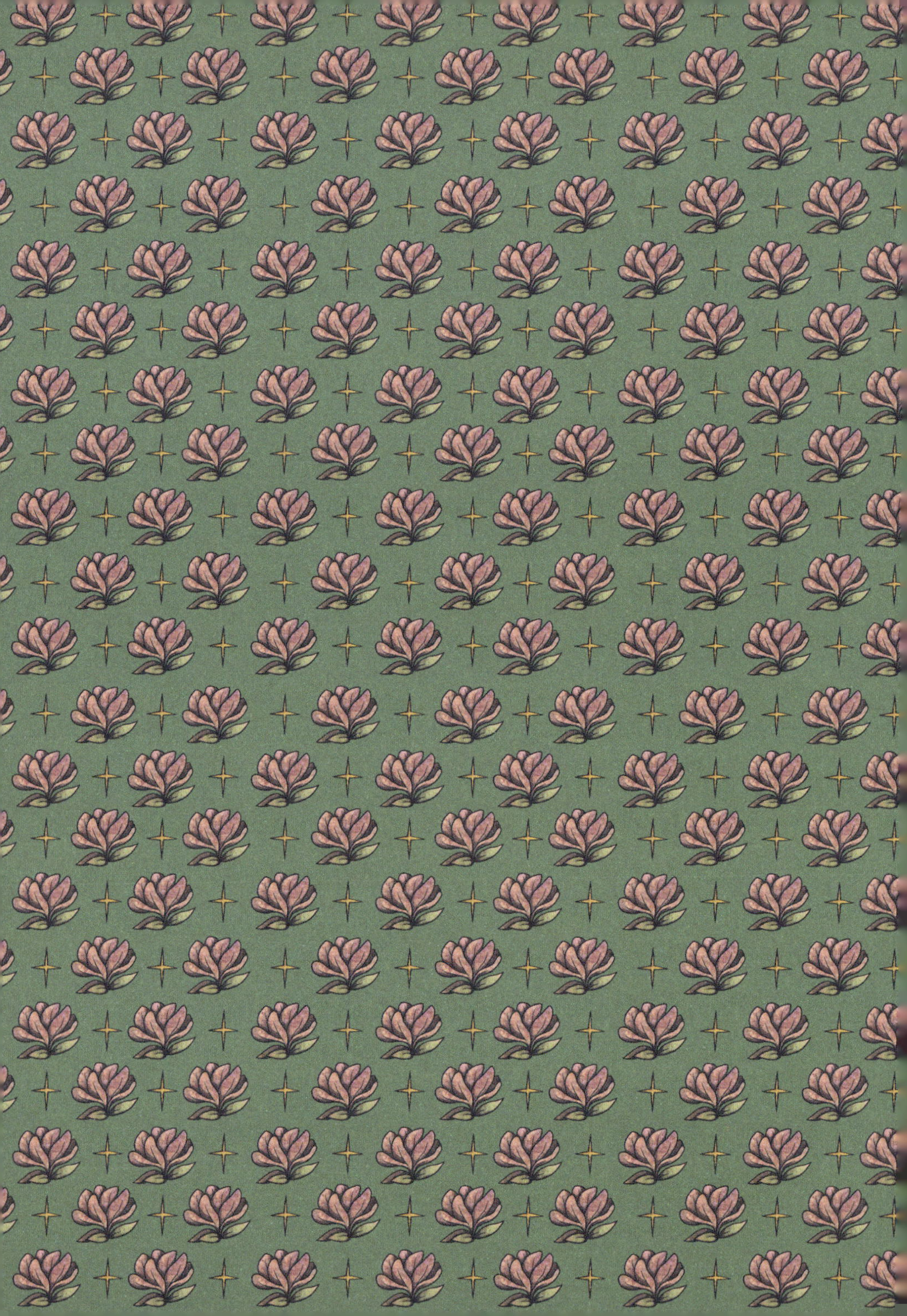